——Dr. Zhong's——
PEDIATRIC
ESSENTIALS

——— Dr. Zhong's ———
PEDIATRIC ESSENTIALS

A Clinical Guide for Treating Children in
the Traditional Chinese Medicine Clinic

Dr. Zhong Bai Song PhD, LAc

Edited by Michael Johnston L.Ac., M.S.O.M.

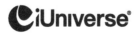

DR. ZHONG'S PEDIATRIC ESSENTIALS
A Clinical Guide for Treating Children in the
Traditional Chinese Medicine Clinic

iUniverse books may be ordered through booksellers or by contacting:

iUniverse
1663 Liberty Drive
Bloomington, IN 47403
www.iuniverse.com
1-800-Authors (1-800-288-4677)

ISBN: 978-1-4917-9704-4 (sc)
ISBN: 978-1-4917-9703-7 (e)

Library of Congress Control Number: 2016907746

Print information available on the last page.

iUniverse rev. date: 06/22/2016

CONTENTS

PREFACE

After learning, practicing, researching and teaching TCM pediatrics for more than 30 years I decided to publish this book based on my experience. I obtained my Bachelor of medicine in Luzhou Medical College, and Master's degree after studying with one of China's most famous TCM pediatricians, Professor Xiao Zhengan. Then I obtained my Ph.D. studying with one of the most prominent physicians of integrative pediatric and internal medicine in Sichuan Province, Dr. Wu Kangheng. I have read most of the TCM classics in Chinese and current TCM pediatrics works in English. I feel there are not many works that broadly and deeply introduce TCM pediatrics in theory and practice. This is why I have spent the last seven years writing this book. In this book, we will do our best to introduce TCM pediatrics integrating the following:

(1) Classical theory and clinical experience of TCM pediatrics.
(2) Theory of the classics, current TCM and Western medical science.
(3) Classic diseases as well as modern diseases that have occurred in recent years. Emphasis was put on the classic diseases, but we will explore modern diseases and how they pertain to TCM pediatric theory.
(4) Treatment and prevention of disease.
(5) Treatments using medication and non-drug therapies. Classical TCM therapy is introduced, while traditional non-drug therapies, such as acupuncture, Tuina, topical therapy and the author's experience also are introduced.

I sincerely thank those who made significant contributions to this book without your help and dedication this project would not have been possible. Many thanks to Marie Fruchenicht L.Ac, Sameul Leong L.Ac., Gregory Sparkman L.Ac., Dr. Benjamin Hsu, Jianyi Hou, Lily Yang and Stella M. Stoufer.

A Brief History of Pediatrics of TCM

TCM pediatrics is a clinical science that researches the growth, development, nursing, conservation, prevention and therapy of children's diseases within the context of Traditional Chinese medicine. It has a rich history, medical books and records reliably document the early identification of diseases and their therapies.

Bian Que was the first pediatrician in Chinese history. Historical records dating (104-91 BCE) state that "The medical techniques of Bian Que were legendary. He went to Xian Yang where people love children, and became a pediatrician."

The earliest children's medical records were written by Chun Yu Yin based on his clinical experience. There were records about pediatrics in many other medical books as well. The Huang Di Nei Jing Su Wen (Yellow Emperor's Canon on Internal Medicine and the Plain Questions) on vacuity and repletion states: "The Yellow Emperor asked Qi Bo when one has just given birth to a baby and contracts fever with a very tiny pulse, what does it imply?" Qi Bo replied "the patient may survive when his feet are warm, and will die when his feet are cold." The Yellow Emperor asked "if a baby is attacked by wind-heat with the symptom of making sounds during respiration, opening his mouth and lifting his shoulders to breathe, what will happen to him?" Qi Bo said "when his pulse is floating and slow, he may survive; if his pulse is rapid, he will die." The Su Wen on extraordinary diseases states: "Some people have epilepsy since they were born, what is this disease and how does it come about?" Qi Bo said "it is called infantile epilepsy, it happens because the mother became severely frightened while the baby was still in her womb, her Qi reversed upwards and failed to come down, and the assembling of the fright caused the baby to have epilepsy when he was born." In a section of the Ling Shu (The Spiritual Pivot) titled Determine the Disease by Taking Pulse states: "When an infant has a disease with his hair standing upward, he will die. If he has a green vein bulging around his ear, it shows he has spasm pain." The Ling Shu on the progress of overweight and slim physiques states "The muscles of an infant are soft, he has little blood and his Qi is weaker". All of these books have information related to the physiology and pulse of children. In 1972 volumes of silk scrolls were discovered at an archeological site in Ma Wang Dui in Hunan province. This tomb was originally sealed in 168 BCE. Among the many documents found there, were nineteen volumes of formulas for women and children in the *Han Shu Yi Wen Zhi* (The Treatise on Literature) in 32-92 BCE. These records included information on kids suffering from seizures and convulsions. All of the above, and more, are considered to be the writings that formed the beginnings of TCM pediatrics. With the developments in society and TCM, during the Jin, Sui, and Tang dynasties (3rd -10th Centuries) TCM pediatrics followed a certain protocol. The children's diseases were put into categories, and there were more than 100 formulas created for children. There were abundant theories on pediatric health, which were more applicable. There are six volumes of pediatrics in the *Zhu Bing Yuan Huo Lun* (General Treatise on the Causes and symptoms of diseases) by Chao Yuan-fang in 610B.C. and this discussed 255 syndromes of children. It also talked about children's nursing and the etiology of diseases in detail. There are nine chapters about pediatric diseases and 325 formulas in the *Bie Ji Qian Jin Yao Fang* (Thousand Ducat Formulas) by Sun Si Miao in 652 CE. Dr. Wang Tao in his book, *Wai Tai Mi Yao* (Secret and Importance of Medicine) in 752 CE puts the children's syndromes into 86 categories and records 400 formulas for pediatrics.

At the end of the Tang dynasty, the earliest known book on TCM pediatrics was written, *Lu Xin Jing* (Classic of Fontanel). This book first characterized a child's constitution as pure yang. This book also discusses methods of pulse taking and therapies to treat convulsions, epilepsy, malnutrition and dysentery. The Medical

Education Bureau was created by the national government during the Tang dynasty, 618-907. There were five departments, internal medicine, surgery, pediatrics, ENT and Tuina. After the students completed medical school and passed their exams they interned with medical doctors for five years. At that point they would choose a specialty such as pediatrics. These were the pioneers of pediatrics.

The Formation of TCM Pediatrics

With the development of scientific techniques during the Song dynasty (960~1279), there were many experts and specialized subjects regarding pediatrics, which became the foundation of TCM pediatrics. In the Song dynasty, there were many works that discussed the characteristics of pediatrics, such as the features of physiology, pathology, diagnosis and treatment.

The main developments include the following:

- The diagnostic methods of Pediatrics Zang Fu differentiation were established.
- The diagnostic methods unique to Pediatrics were developed. Observations of the face and index vein were covered.
- The therapies in pediatrics were rich and colorful. Xiao Er Yue Zheng Zhi Jue (The Keys to Differentiation and Treatment of Children's Diseases) comprehensively points out the theories of TCM pediatrics.

Dr. Qian Yi (1032~1113) made the following contributions to TCM pediatrics:

- Dr. Qian summarized the children's physiological features of the Zang and Fu organs as fragile, immature and imperfect, and their pathological features as Yi Xu Yi Shi (being subject to vacuity and repletion) and Yi Han Yi Re (being subject to cold and heat).
- He focused on inspection within the four diagnostics of TCM, especially on the signs of complexion and eyes.

3

- He founded the pediatric differentiation principles of the Zang Fu, and created formulas such as Xie Bai San (Purge the White Powder), Xie Huang San (Purge the Yellow Powder), Dao Chi San (Guide the Red Powder), Xie Qing Wan (Purge the Green Powder) and Liu Wei Di Huang Wan (Six-ingredient pill with rehmannia) these formulas remain clinically effective today.
- He discussed measles, smallpox, convulsions and malnutrition. These were considered the four difficult diseases in ancient China. He also distinguished among measles, smallpox and chickenpox.
- He advocated treating acute and chronic convulsions differently. He suggested that acute convulsions should be treated by cooling and purging, and chronic convulsions by warming and supplementing.

He summarized all malnutrition diseases as disorders of the spleen and stomach, due to yin, blood and body fluid damage. Dr. Qian Yi and his work became the foundation of TCM pediatrics. Measles and smallpox spread widely in the Song dynasty. There was academic debate about how to treat them with either warming or cooling therapies. The earliest monograph for smallpox and measles were written by Dr. Dong Ji in his work *Xiao Er Ban Zhen Bei Ji Fang Lun* (Pediatric Macula and Rashes for Emergency) in 1093. In this book he wrote that it is good to treat warm disorders related to the macula and rashes with cold and cool herbs, such as Bai Hu Tang (White Tiger Decoction), he warned against the use of warming and supplementing herbs for these kinds of issues. Later on, Dr. Cheng Wen Zhong, in 1251, boldly used the warm and replenishing herbs for warm disorders related to macula and rashes. He found that Fu Zi (radix aconiti carmichaeli) and Rou Gui (cinnamon bark) were useful for these disorders when they were due to yang exhaustion. There were many more developments in other pediatric works about pediatrics' unique diagnostic qualities, inspection of the index vein, surgery, therapy, and preventive medicine all related to children. For example, in the book *You You Xin Shu* (New Pediatrics), in 1330 the unique diagnostic method of inspecting the index vein was founded. In the *Xiao Er Wei Sheng Zhong Wei Fan Lun* (General Hygiene of Pediatrics) in 1156, eleven shapes of the index vein were recorded. It discussed many hereditary malformations, such as cleft palate, syndactyly, polydactyly, renal agenesis, and dwarfism. His book introduced some surgical operations for cleft palate, syndactyly, polydactyly and abnormal fingers. This book also recognized that newborn tetanus is the same disease as adult tetanus, and that this was due to incorrect cutting of the umbilical cord with a cold knife. He recommended using moxa to burn the umbilical cord of a newborn in order to prevent tetanus, and putting herbs on the umbilicus. This is an effective way to prevent tetanus in newborns and he created topical therapies to help children.

Development of TCM Pediatrics

TCM pediatrics became more refined during the Jin (1115~1234), Yuan (1271~1368), Ming (1368~1644) and Qing (1636~1912) dynasties. Dr. Wan Quan put forward the school of children's tendency to vacuity of the lungs, spleen and kidneys, and surplus of the heart and liver in his three works, *Yu Ying Jia Mi* (Family Secret for Children's Conservation), 1541, *Pian Yu Xin Shu* (Piece of Experience of Pediatrics) 1578, and *You Ke Fa Hui* (Education of Pediatrics) 1579. These help to explain the characteristics of pediatric pathology and diagnosis. Dr. Wu Tang in his work *Wen Bing Tiao Bian Jie Er Nan* (Difficulties in Pediatrics of Differentiation of Warm Febrile Disease) states when children are less than 3 years of age their young yang and their young yin is vulnerable. This becomes the doctrine of pure yang, and the foundational theory of TCM pediatrics. Dr. Ye Tian Shi set forth the protocols for differentiating the warm disease according to four levels. His doctrine helped pediatric diagnostic methods in clinic become more effective. In his book, *Lin Zheng Zhi Nan Yi An Jie Er Nan* (Case Records as a Guide to Clinical Practice fn Difficulties in Pediatrics) he put forward "For children, they tend to have heat syndromes because of their pure yang constitution." Since then, the diagnosis and therapies for internal miscellaneous diseases of children follow the differentiation and therapies of the five Zang, while warm febrile diseases of children utilize the framework of Wei, Qi, Ying and blood differentiation.

Pediatric preventive medicine during this period also had outstanding achievements. Physicians Xue Kai and Xue Ji in their book, *Bao Yin Chuo Yao* (Conservation and Importance for Children), 1505, introduced "burning down the umbilicus" to prevent newborn tetanus. This work dramatically decreased the cases of newborn tetanus. Methods to prevent smallpox were focused upon, and much progress was made in this field. Human inoculations were recorded in the *Bo Ji Xi Dou Fang* (The Methods of Wide Dilution of Smallpox)1577, and the *Zhong Dou Xin Shu* (New Book of Inoculation), 1741, as well as in the *Zhong Dou Xin Fa* (New Way of Inoculation), 1808.

There were a lot of specialized books on measles published. For example, *Ma Ke Huo Ren Quan Shu* (The Comprehensive Book Specializing in Measles and Life Rescue) 1748. This book discussed the differentiation of measles, the sequelae and complications of measles. The *Ma Zhen Ji Cheng* (Comprehensive Measles), 1879, discussed the indication and contraindications of diet and herbal formulas for measles. A lot of pediatric works published enriched the pediatric theories and clinical practices. For instance, *Bao Yin Chuo Yao* (Conservation Importance for Children) 1505, discussed many children's internal diseases. It also put forward the idea of "preventing children's disorders by educating nursing mothers, and treating both the mother and child when children become sick". Dr. Wan Quan focused on protecting the spleen and stomach in his three books *Yu Ying Jia Mi* (Family secret for Children's Conservation) 1541, *Pian Yu Xin Shu* (Pieces of Experience in Pediatrics) 1578, and *You Ke Fa Hui* (Education of Pediatrics) 1579. Xia Yu Xi focused on observing the complexion and orifices of children in his book *You Ke Tie Jing* (Iron Mirror for pediatrics) 1695, which can help differentiate between patterns of cold, heat, vacuity and repletion of the zang and fu. He also invented the burning therapy (Deng Huo Liao Fa) for newborn tetanus.

Pediatric Tuina plays an important role in children's health. Pediatric manipulation is different from adult manipulation. In the beginning it was considered a kind of myth. However, the theory took shape systematically during the Ming and Qing dynasties.

There were many pediatric Tuina works published during these periods. For example, Dr. Gong Yun Lin'work, *Xiao Er Tui Na Fang Mai Huo Ying Mi Zhi* (Pediatric Tui Na and TCM for Rescuing Life) 1604. In 1605 Zhuo Yu Fan wrote *Xiao Er Tui Na Mi Jue* (Secrets of Pediatric Tui Na,). Xiong Ying Xiong's wrote *Tui Na Guang Yi* (Wider Meaning of Tui Na) in 1676. Zhang Zhen Yun wrote *Li Zheng An Mo Yao Shu* (Corrected and Important Techniques of Tui Na) 1888.

Characteristics of Pediatric Physiology and Pathology

In humans, children are not only different in their physical makeup and physiology, but also in their incidence of diseases in terms of disease types and disease development. Grasping the differences in physiological and pathological characteristics between children and adults is important for proper clinical diagnosis, treatment and care. Physicians began to understand children's characteristics in the *Huang Di Nei Jing* (Yellow Emperor's Canon of Internal Medicine). This formed a relatively complete set of physiological and pathological features through the efforts of those contemporary physicians. The primary characteristics in ancient times were Pure Yang (Chun Yang), Young Yin (Zhi Yin) and Young Yang (Zhi Yang). It was said "children are easy to have vacuity and easy to have repletion, easy to have cold and easy to have heat". Their characteristics are accurately summarized as delicate zang and fu, immature physique, vigorous vitality, rapid growth and development, easy onset and rapid transformation, clear and agile zang qi and easy rehabilitation.

Physiological Characteristics

A new born child is a sprout. From birth to adulthood, humans are in a continuous process of growth and development. The main difference in this process between children and adults is that things occur much more quickly and significantly in children. Therefore we cannot just say that children are little adults.

Delicate Zang and Fu, Immature Physique and Qi

Zang and fu refer to the five zang and six fu organs. Physique refers to the constitution and configuration of the human body and its essence, blood and other body fluids. Qi refers to all physiological functions of the body. In childhood, regardless of their physical structure, their zang and fu organs are fragile, and their functional activities are immature and imperfect. These vulnerabilities are more significant at the younger ages. The *Ling Shu* (Spiritual Pivot) stated, "Children's flesh is fragile, their blood is scanty, and their Qi is weak." It went on to say, "The child's blood is not sufficient; their gastrointestinal tracts are vulnerable; their Qi is cowardly, their spines are soft and weak; their fontanelles are not closed, and they can't stand up." The teeth are considered the excess of the bone, they come in stages, so the children will chew unevenly. The brain hasn't developed; therefore, they act cowardly, cry easily, and their actions are very dynamic. The skin is soft and easily penetrable; their defensive Qi (Wei Qi) is weak, and they are susceptible to invasion from external pathogens. Their gastrointestinal tracts are immature and digestive problems form easily. Therefore, ancient physicians summarized the characteristics of children as young Yin and young Yang (Zhi Yin Zhi Yang) which is to say that in children, both Yin, physical makeup, and Yang, functional activities, are peurile, imperfect and continuously changeable.

Vigorous in Vitality, Rapid Growth and Development

Children are in a period of continuous growth and development. The younger the child is, the faster these changes happen. Their vitality is exuberant, and changes come on very rapidly. The height, weight, cranial circumference, thoracic circumference, teeth and fontanel closure of a one-year-child change in every month. For example, the weight of a one-year-child is three times greater than that of a newborn. The height is one and a half times greater, and the cranial circumference increases by 50%. Their actions, language, intelligence, and zang fu function at this age can also change rapidly as they move towards maturity. Ancient physicians said Pure Yang (Chun Yang) can be summarized in this way: "As

9

children begin to thrive they are exuberant and vigorous in their growth, just like a plant sprouting or the sun rising in the eastern sky. Pure Yang should not be considered as excessive yang with vacuity of yin or yang without yin."

Pathological Characteristics

Children's physiological characteristics are different from those of an adult. Therefore, the onset, types of diseases, and evolution of diseases in children are quite different.

Easy Onset and Rapid Transformation

A child's physiological characteristics include two primary features. Children are easily affected by invasion of the six pathogenic factors and they are also vulnerable to disorders of the lung, spleen, stomach, and kidneys. After the onset of disease, transformation typically happens quite rapidly. There can be repletion or vacuity, cold or heat, and mixed combinations of repletion, vacuity, cold, and heat. Children's pathological features are summarized as "Yi Xu Yi Shi" (being subject to vacuity and repletion) and "Yi Han Yi Re"(being subject to cold and heat). Yi Xu Yi Shi means that once a child is ill, pathogenic factors are easy to become excessive while the qi is weak. Repletion syndromes may easily change into vacuity, or we may see a mixed syndrome of repletion and vacuity in a relatively short period of time. Yi Han Yi Re means that the child is easy to have heat syndromes because their constitution is Pure Yang and Young Yin. They are also susceptible to cold syndromes because of their Young Yang. Furthermore, their cold or heat condition may quickly transform into the other or show a syndrome with mixed heat and cold. For example, a child can easily have a cold with a cough due to exterior wind. If it is not treated properly, this can quickly become pneumonia with a high fever, cough, dyspnea, phlegm, and flaring of the nostrils, which is a replete heat syndrome. Meanwhile, this weak qi cannot overcome these pathogenic factors. This excessive heat may evolve into a critical situation such as heart yang vacuity or even collapse of the heart yang manifested with a pale and purple appearance, cold extremities and cold sweating, a deep and weak pulse, and shortness of breath

Clear and Agile Zang Qi, Easy Rehabilitation

Even though children's diseases come on easily and transform rapidly, a child's zang fu organs have a strong ability to heal because of their robust vitality. Etiology in children is relatively simple. They are mainly affected by the six exogenous pathogenic factors, warm febrile pathogens, and dietary disorders. Children suffer less from chronic and stubborn illnesses. In addition, they have less emotional interference. Their response to therapy has a higher sensitivity because their zang qi is clear, agile, and effective. Children recover more easily from diseases than adults if they are diagnosed correctly and treated promptly. In the pediatric chapter of Dr. Zhang Jing Nue's book, *Jing Yue Encyclopedia,* he says, "Children's zang qi is clear and agile, and will respond immediately when doctors treat them. Their diseases can be cured in one treatment as long as doctors accurately understand the root of the disease. This is not true in adults who suffer from more recalcitrant diseases."

Pure Yang, Young Yin and Young Yang

Pure Yang (Chun Yang)

The younger the child is, the more vigorous they will be in their vitality, growth, and development. This is referred to as Pure Yang (Chun Yang). This is a major feature of the child's constitution. It is also pointed out in the *Lu Xin Jing* (The Classics of Skull and Fontanelle) 25-220, that in children who are younger than three years old, Yuan Qi is still in their body. It is termed Pure Yang (Chun Yang). In Feng Shi's chapter, Acute Convulsion of Children he states, "Tian Gui means Yin Qi. A child is considered pure Yang because his Yin Qi is insufficient". By Pure Yang, in terms of physiology, it is meant that Yang is abundant compared to Yin which is insufficient comparatively. Physiologically, Pure Yang is defined as having vigorous vitality and rapid growth and development. Dr. Ye Tian Shi, in his book Essentials of Pediatrics stated, "The diseases that most children contract belong to heat patterns because their constitution is pure Yang. Once ill, especially with infants and toddlers, their diseases are easy to change to heat and fire syndromes, even stirring up wind. This explains why children's diseases are mostly heat-oriented and typically include high fever, convulsions, and unconsciousness. Moreover, children recover faster and more easily from diseases than adults. These are the pathological characteristics of Pure Yang.

Young Yin and Young Yang (Zhi Yin and Zhi Yang)

Zhi means puerile, tender, immature, and imperfect yin, in this case, refers to the five zang and six fu organs, the constitution and configuration of the human body, and its essence, blood, and body fluids. Yang refers to the physiological functions of the zang fu organs. *Wen Bing Tiao Bia Jie Er Nan* (Difficulties in Pediatrics of Differentiation of Warm Febrile Diseases) states: "Children's young yang is insufficient, and their young yin is imperfect." Current physicians consider the so-called "delicate zang and fu" and "immature physique and qi" as the Young Yin and Young Yang. "Easy onset and rapid transformation" is a statement referring to the pathological state common in children due to the weakness of their defensive qi causing them to become ill more easily than adults. Once the onset of an illness occurs, it will rapidly transform between repletion and vacuity, cold and heat, or a mixed syndrome.

The doctrine of children as "Pure Yang" and "Young Yin and Young Yang" is a primary characteristic in pediatric medicine which continues to evolve with the development of Chinese medicine. They have their own meanings and different physiological and pathological significance. Pure Yang refers to a child's potential for growth and development which is fueled by an abundance of yang qi. It is not considered to be repletion of yang or a vacuity of yin, it is a normal condition. The Young Yin and Young Yang refer to the inherent imperfection and immaturity in a child's constitution. Young Yin and Young Yang are dependent upon Pure Yang in order for the child to reach maturity. Pure Yang is both full of vigor and vitality and at the same time is immature and wild. Physiologically it is the catalyst for a child's rapid growth and development, pathologically it allows for rapid onset and development of disease patterns that are typically hot in nature; disease patterns that can quickly consume immature yin. The *Su Wen* states: "there is yang qi in humans like there is a sun in the sky. When the sun is not in its proper position the heavens and earth will become dark and when the yang qi of the man is not in the proper position he will die early." Yang is the driving force of life and it is the main force of resistance. In children, we must have a comprehensive understanding of how this complex interplay of yin and yang exist pathologically and physiologically in order to best prevent and control disease processes and ensure healthy growth. Therefore, the doctrine of Pure Yang, Young Yin and Young Yang completely explain the physical characteristics of children and is one of Chinese medicine's guiding principles.

Characteristics of the Five Zang Organs

A famous pediatrician, Wan Quan, (Ming Dynasty 1368-1644) pointed out that in a child's zang organs "the liver has a surplus, the spleen is insufficient, the kidneys are commonly vacuous, heart fire and liver fire are similar, the lungs are tender and are easy to be injured and difficult to cure." The lungs, spleen and kidney are insufficient while the liver and heart have a surplus. Dr. Wan Quan went on to say "the surpluses and insufficiencies do not mean vacuity or repletion pathologically", it mainly refers to Pure Yang, Young Yin, Young Yang of the five zang organs in terms of their relative performance.

The Liver is commonly in Surplus

The methods for supplementing yin and reducing for repletion and vacuity of the five zang organs in *You Ke Fa Hui* (Elaborating on Pediatrics) pointed out: "The liver is commonly in surplus, because the liver's qi is Shao Yang. Human beings are born just like sprouts of grasses and wood, which is the Shao Yang qi, growing up and becoming gradually stronger and stronger, so there is surplus". The constitution of children is Pure Yang like the beginning of a new year or the growth of a new tree. There is an abundance of potential energy. It is the natural surplus of vigorous growth that is the qi of Shao Yang and the liver is the wood phase. This is the physiological meaning of the liver being in surplus. The pathological significance is that children tend to have hyperactivity of the liver and stirring of the liver qi when they become sick.

The Spleen is Commonly Insufficient

This concept is significant in two ways. First, a child's spleen and stomach are immature in their form and function. Second, their rapid growth and development demand more nutrition. Therefore, in comparison between the shape and quality of the pediatric spleen/stomach and the nutritional needs for optimal growth, their imperfections are much clearer and their immaturity is easily recognizable. This common insufficiency should never be counted as a general vacuity or pathological, it is simply the tendency of the pediatric spleen and stomach.

The pathological significance is that the spleen qi in a child is not robust and that the stomach is small and tender and cannot contain large amounts of food. Therefore, it is crucial for a child's nutrition to be appropriate for their age and size. If patients are nursed and fed even slightly inappropriately, the spleen and stomach may be easily damaged. This will result in failure of the spleen and stomach to generate qi and blood. Eventually this may lead to many diseases and ultimately to abnormal growth and development. When we practice pediatric care close attention must be paid these facts.

The Kidney is commonly vacuous

The Universal Truth of Plain Questions said "For a woman, her kidney energy becomes prosperous when she is seven, her milk teeth fall off and the permanent teeth emerge. Her Tian Gui appears at the age of fourteen. At this time, her Ren channel begins to put through, and her Chong channel becomes prosperous and her menstruation begins to appear. She can be pregnant and bear a child. For a man, his kidney energy becomes prosperous by the age of eight., his hair develops and his permanent teeth emerge. His kidney energy becomes prosperous by the age of sixteen. If he conducts sexual intercourse with a woman, he may have a child." Wan Quan also said "the kidney is in charge of vacuity, which refers to insufficiency." This refers to both the yin and yang of the children's kidney, that they are not full and that they are physiologically immature. Just as many classics have said "the kidney does not have repletion syndromes". Thus, we have to pay attention to supplement and take care of the children's kidney yin and yang in order to ensure minimal depletion and offer them the best chance at gradual and complete maturity.

The Heart is commonly replete

The heart belongs to fire and yang. The constitution of the child is also yang. Therefore, physiologically, their heart fire and yang are comparatively and naturally in surplus. Pathologically, the fire of the heart tends to stirring up especially during warm, febrile diseases.

The Lung is delicate and tender

In physiology, the lung is more tender than the other zang organs. The lung does not receive adequate qi from the spleen as the spleen is the mother of the lung, and a child's spleen is immature. Therefore, the lung is particularly fragile. This causes children to be more prone to suffering from respiratory diseases that can be difficult to cure. In the clinic, pediatric pulmonary diseases occur frequently and can be critical and intractable. The success of their treatment is easily affected by their diet, daily life and other factors.

Chinese medicine considers the lung, spleen and kidney to have the closest relationship with the vital Qi (Zheng Qi). This is because the lung governs the qi, the spleen is the acquired foundation and the kidney is the inherited foundation. The main function of the Zheng Qi is defense which is referenced in the *Su Wen* as "evil Qi will not invade when the vital Qi is sufficient and the evil Qi will invade when the vital Qi is insufficient." The vital

Qi and defensive Qi in children are insufficient and immature. This causes children to become sick easier than adults, and most of these illnesses will belong to patterns of the lung, spleen and kidney.

The Main Factors Determining an Individual Constitution

In clinic, there are not only many differences in children among their height, weight, preference for cold or heat, dietary habits and personality at the same age, but also in the ways they may or may not contract diseases. Some will tend to cold patterns, some to hot. Some may heal easily while others' illnesses are more recalcitrant. Two children may have different reactions to the same treatment. All of these factors are related to their constitution in TCM and this can be due to several reasons.

The constitution in ancient TCM books was described as "the quality of the inherited body", "intrinsic elements of body", "intrinsic quality" and many other expressions. It refers to an individual whose different nationality and groups format a comparative stability between the growth and decline of yin and yang, the static and dynamic trends, and manifestations of the inherent characteristics in the morphology and physiological functions. This is decided by various inherited and acquired factors. This feature often contains certain risk factors which determine their susceptibility and pathological types of bias. Therefore, it has great significance for us to understand physical characteristics and individual constitutions of children. In addition we must recognize important factors in the formation of individual differences in the well child.

According to ancient and modern TCM Pediatrics there are two primary factors which determine one's constitution.

- Inherited Factors
  The formation of different physical constitutions in children is related to many factors, but the most important ones being inherited. Bing (稟), in Chinese means natural endowment, Fu (賦) means giving. Ancient doctors said "infants are given everything by their parents before they

are born". So "what can make infants develop robustly and strong with good physical balance is something that starts at the beginning of the pregnancy, not after they are born".

- Postnatal Factors
  Ancient physicians said "children may have a long life if they are nurtured properly, even if they are born with a poor constitution. They may have many severe diseases and die young even though they have a strong constitution." This means that postnatal factors play a crucial role that can either support or conflict with a child's genetic makeup.

The influence of the diet

This is one of the most obvious influences upon a child's constitution. It is beneficial to the child's health to eat a nutritious and balanced diet. The *Shu Wen Zang Qi Fa Shi* (Plain Questions on zang fu and time effect) states "five kinds of rice can nourish the body, five kinds of fruits can generate body, five kinds of animals can enrich the body, and five kinds of vegetables can supplement the body." This statement means that a nutritious and varied diet is crucial, and it is important to avoid certain foods and not over do it, because "overfeeding of sweet may cause malnutrition, over fullness may damage qi, over cold food causes food stagnation, over sour damages zhi, over bitter consumes shen, over salty closes qi, over greasy produces phlegm, over pungent injures the lung." All of these indicate that the desire for one kind of food may affect the constitution and lead, finally, to illness.

The Influence of Living

As early as the 6th and 7th centuries, ancient physicians in the Sui (589-618) and Tang (618-907) dynasties knew children's constitutions were affected by daily life. It is important for children to become strong and to balance their constitution. "When the weather is fine and without strong wind, parents should hold their children and play outside. If they do so often, this will increase the child's defensive function and help to prevent disease. It will

17

build up their Qi and blood and strengthen their muscles. On the other hand, if children are always kept inside and overdressed, they cannot develop a defense mechanism to external pathogenic factors; just like grass growing in a damp and dark place without enough sunshine will be delicate and easy to die." This was stated in the *Zhu Bing Yuan Hou Lun* (General Treatise on the Causes and symptoms of diseases) 610. Dr. Chen Wen Zhong, in his book, *Xiao Er Bing Yuan Fang Lun* (The Courses of Diseases in Pediatrics) 1254 CE, suggests ten nursing methods: "the back, abdomen and feet should keep warm. The head, chest and heart should keep cool, avoid seeing monsters. One should keep the spleen and stomach warm. Don't take medicine that has severe side effects or heavy metal, such as cinnabar and lead."

The Influence of Diseases and Medicine

Diseases and medicine may lead to an imbalance between the root Yin and Yang, which in turn may change the balance in our day to day health. If this problem becomes chronic then it will then create imbalance in the constitution. It is more obvious in childhood. As children's bodies are delicate, if they suffer some disease for a protracted time, damage can easily occur. For example, a child who experiences prolonged vomiting with fever will easily suffer damage to their yin. If this goes on uncorrected, over time their constitution will now include this component of yin vacuity. This often happens with children who are treated incorrectly or are given excessive dosages over long periods of time. Jing stated "The qi and blood of the child is insufficient. It is most important for children to be nourished properly, and to use medications with caution."

Development, Growth and Care

A child's constitution, physiological function, body movement, language and intelligence are constantly changing as they develop from the time they are born. This affects their pathological features. It is very important to understand this idea when considering how to nurse and care for them, treat them with medicine and most importantly prevent illness.

It is important to understand the growth and developmental characteristics of age and stages during childhood.

Gestational Stage-The First 40 weeks

The fetus in utero relies entirely upon its mother for survival. The growth and development of the fetus is influenced by the mother's diet, daily work, rest, emotional state and so on. Malnutrition, emotional disorders, drugs, smoking, alcohol, radiation, environmental pollution or maternal disease can lead to fetal retardation, miscarriage, premature birth, birth defects, and ultimately still birth.

Parents must begin nourishing, protecting and educating the fetus as soon as the pregnancy is discovered. The fetus is directly or indirectly influenced by the internal and external environment. Nourishing the fetus means that the pregnant woman has sufficient nutrition utilizing the "five flavors". This refers to a diet that includes a variety of foods that will ensure proper balance and offer the most nutrients. Protection of the fetus means that the pregnant woman will properly balance work and rest. This will help to maintain robust health and minimize suffering during the pregnancy. Fetal education means that the mother will strive to keep her spirit strong for the benefit of the fetus. She should avoid "seeing the bad colors" and "hearing the violent music". In other words she should try to create an internal environment for the fetus which is positive and glorious. If she keeps the external environment free from negative influence, this will echo internally and benefit the developing child.

Neonatal stage- Birth to 28 days

Newborn infants, especially in the first week of birth have a high incidence of mortality because the baby has undergone great changes in their external environment, physiological functions, and their ability to adapt is weak. The diseases during this period are mostly related with intrauterine retardation, birth trauma, asphyxia, congenital malformations and infections. While a variety of problems may potentially occur, they may not present with typical clinical manifestation; thus practitioners should try to get all the information about the patient.

In order to help newborn infants grow and develop in a healthy way, ancient physicians created methods to care for them, such as how to swab the infant's mouth, how to bathe them, how to cut and care for the umbilicus, how to expel internal toxins, how to breastfeed and how to clothe them.

Infancy Stage- Day 29 to Day 365

Infancy is the stage of the fastest growth and development in a human life. Their weight may increase by 2-3 times by the time they are one year old. Their height will increase by double or more, their head will grow to 12 centimeters, and deciduous teeth will emerge.

Infants often suffer from digestive disorders and infections. They demand more nutrients in order to keep up with their rapid growth and development. For example, one kilogram of body weight in an adult requires one gram per day of protein, an infant requires 3.5 grams of protein. The spleen is commonly insufficient;

therefore correct nursing during this period is crucial. If an infant is fed inappropriately, their spleen and stomach can become easily damaged. This results in the stomach and spleen failing to generate qi and blood, leading to such diseases as anemia, malnutrition, 5 delays and 5 weaknesses syndrome.

The infant's immune function that was inherited from the mother will gradually disappear within about 6 months. As the parents begin to take the infant outside more and more the child will be vulnerable to contraction of external pathogenic factors causing warm febrile and respiratory diseases that can turn to fire and cause stirring of internal wind.

The most important factor in terms of nursing and feeding is selecting nutrition that will satisfy their needs during this time of rapid growth and development and is in accordance with the physiological characteristics of an infant's spleen and stomach. Breastfeeding is strongly encouraged with weaning to begin at around 9 or 10 months. This can be done earlier or later based on a family's specific circumstances. Gradually add supplementation before weaning in order to meet the baby's nutritional needs and to train the baby to eat meals at regular times.

Create a good environment for the baby. Try to keep the baby's bowel movements smooth and make sure they get the rest they need. Parents should pay close attention to their child's development.

Toddler Stage- Age 1 to 3

The toddler years are a time of great cognitive and emotional development and when social and language skills begin to develop. Change may occur as a result of genetic processes known as maturation or they may be due to environmental factors and what is learned through adult contact. Their anterior fontanels are fully closed after 18 months. As the bones of the skull thicken, 16 deciduous teeth will nearly be finished growing. Most toddlers will be able to control their bowel movements and urination by this time. The highest incidents of diseases in toddlers are warm diseases and pulmonary diseases such as cough, pneumonia, and asthma. The second highest incidences of diseases are disorders of the spleen and stomach such as poor appetite, vomiting, and diarrhea. It is necessary for toddlers to have good dietary habits and good nutrition in order to promote an active and healthy lifestyle. Close attention should be paid to providing clothing that is appropriate for the season and changing weather patterns. Vaccinations can help prevent infectious diseases.

The Preschool Stage- Age 3 to 7

In this period their increases in weight and height are slower than the previous period. But their language and behavioral skills increase dramatically. They have high energy and are very active during this time. In addition to the diseases mentioned above, children at this stage also have higher incidence of accidental injury, poisoning, and diseases related to the immune system such as asthma, juvenile rheumatoid arthritis and nephritis.

The characteristics of feeding in this period resemble the habits of an adult rather than a toddler. Important points include:

- offer a balanced and healthy diet
- train the preschooler to eat proper portions
- monitor their height and weight to determine proper nutrition
- increase outdoor activities and physical exercise to increase immunity
- protect their teeth and eyes from illness
- avoid aspiration of foreign bodies
- train them with good habits and customs increase their intelligence through speaking, reading, computing, music and art

School Stage- Age 6 to 14

The development of internal organs and body systems at this stage resembles those of adults such as slower heart rate, increased lung capacity, shedding of deciduous teeth and eruption of permanent teeth. Growth and development of the whole body is in a relatively stable state and the incidences of diseases are like that of adults.

Special concerns in addition to those mentioned above are:

- emphasis on personality and the emotional changes of the child
- educate them to have a good character and strong moral standards
- broaden their intelligence through reading, attention, memory, imagination, logical thinking and comprehension

Girls from ages 12 to 18 and boys from ages 14 up to 20 are considered adolescents

Their growth and development in this period can vary due to individual differences.

They will not only gain weight and height greatly, but their secondary sexual characteristics will begin to become obvious. Females will begin menstruation due to rapid development of the reproductive organs. Boys may experience spermatorrhea. Special care must be taken during puberty in order to ensure strong physical and mental health, and to prevent illness or contraction of sexually oriented diseases.

Key signs of growth and development

Body weight

The child's weight is a key sign of growth. It relates to the fetus's gender and the health of the mother's pregnancy. Newborns may lose up to 9% in the first weeks after birth. They will quickly regain that weight. Below is a formula for calculating the weight in order to evaluate their growth.

Age	Weight Formula (g)
1 to 6 months	Weight = weight at birth + 0.7 x months of age
7 to 12 months	Weight = 7 + 0.5 x months of age - 6
2 to 12 years	8 + 2 x years of age

Height

Body height refers to the length from head to foot. This increases much faster at the younger ages. The height of the newborn infant averages 50 cm. The height in the first year increases by about 25 cm. After the age of 2, children will grow 10cm on average per year until age 12. This formula can be applied: Body Height in cm= 70cm + 7cm× age.

Significant increases or lack of height can be due to congenital factors, acquired constitution, diseases or drugs.

Cranial Circumference

This is the length along the upper edge of the eyebrows and around the occipital protuberance. The head circumference of a newborn is 34 cm on average. It is 42 cm at 6 months old and 46 cm at 1 year old. It grows to 48 cm at 2 years old, 50 cm at 5 years old and 54-58cm at 15 years old, this is close to the cranial circumference of an adult. Cranial circumference and brain development are closely related; A circumference being too great or too small indicates abnormal brain growth.

Chest Circumference

Chest circumference is the length described along the lower edge of the nipple around the chest. The chest perimeter of a newborn is 1-2 cm less than that of the head. The perimeters of the head and chest are almost equal at 1 year old. After this age, the chest perimeter exceeds the cranial circumference. Chest size is related to the development of the lung, the thoracic bones, muscles and subcutaneous fat of the chest. If the chest circumference is too small or too big it indicates abnormal development of the chest or the organs in the chest.

Fontanels

The fontanels include the anterior and occipital fontanels. The anterior fontanel are 1.5-2cm in a newborn infant. It will increase with the infant's development in the first 6 months, then they will gradually become smaller until it closes at 12 to 18 months of age.

Some infant's occipital fontanel will close once the infant is born, others will close within 6-8 weeks after birth. The closing of the fontanels is a positive sign of brain development.

Teeth

There are 20 deciduous teeth in children and 32 permanent teeth. The first tooth will emerge at about 4 to 10 months of age. At one year old there will be 6 to 8 teeth and by two and a half years they should have all 20 deciduous teeth. An easy formula to remember is:

- The number of deciduous teeth = age in months 4-6.

The deciduous teeth are replaced with permanent teeth at about age 6 and one should have all of their permanent teeth by ages 20-30 years old.

Respiration

The respiratory rate is the fastest in our first few months. The respiratory rates are as follows for the various ages.

Age (Months)	Breath rates(/minute)
1~3	45~40
4~6	40~35
6~12	35~30
12~36	30~25

The pulse rate is the highest in our first year. The pulse rates are as follows for the various ages.

Age (years)	Pulse rates(/minute)
<1	160~120
1~3	120~100
3~5	110~90
7~12	90~70

Blood Pressure

The younger we are the lower our blood pressure is under normal conditions. The systolic pressure should not be lower than 75-80 mmHg (9.9~10.7kPa) and no more than 120 mmHg (16.0kPa). Diastolic pressure should be no more that 80 mmHg (10.7kPa). The normal blood pressure in children can be calculated using this formula:

Systolic pressure (mmHg) = 80 + 2 x years of age

Diastolic pressure (mmHg) = systolic pressure × 0.5-.33

Motor Skill Development

Fetal movement in the uterus is the original form of exercise. With the rapid development of the brain in the first years after birth, motor skill development happens in certain ways. The general development of motor skills begins from the top of the body to the bottom and is learned in the order of sitting, standing and walking. Our agility goes from uncoordinated to coordinated, from coarse to fine. The infant's motor skills can be summarized as follows:

- they can raise their head in the first two months
- they can roll over within 4 months
- they can crawl with their hands at 7 months
- they can stand at 10 months
- they can distinguish faces at one year
- they can climb stairs at 2 years
- they can dance with hands and feet at 3~4 years old

Language and Intelligence development

Development of language and intelligence reflects the heart and mental development. The language and intelligence development of infants and young children are as follows:

- In one month they should have improved sleep
- At 2 months they begin smiling more and more

- At 3-4 months they will recognize their mother
- At 5-6 months they will try to grab and hold things
- At 7~8 months they will frequently call out for their mother
- At 9~10 months they will begin to pick up words quickly
- At one year, they will begin to show their dislike of things
- At one and a half years they can effectively imitate things
- At two years they may begin to learn how to use the restroom

In addition to the language and intellectual development of a child being related to their age it is also affected by education and communication with others. Therefore, parents should pay attention to the external environment at home, school and other places at which the child spends time. Any and all of this may affect a child's intellectual development.

Psychological and Behavioral Development

The WHO definition of health not only considers physical health, but also includes psychological and behavioral health. Therefore, children should be educated and evaluated in terms of their psychological health and behavior. This will help to ensure a lifetime of physical and mental health. Their training should be focused on building the memory, logical thinking, self control, having a positive mood, balanced emotions and a good personality. Thus, children will develop good morals, they will study and work more effectively and get along better with others.

Nursing of Children

Infants and toddlers grow quickly during childhood. One common pathological feature that is quite obvious in these stages is spleen vacuity. Therefore, it is necessary for their diet to support their rapid growth and development without further damage to the spleen. The ancient physicians had abundant theories and experience in this matter. Ancient physicians from the Sui and Tang Dynasties have advocated breastfeeding, and created an entire breastfeeding method.

Who is a good candidate for breastfeeding?

A woman who is breastfeeding must be healthy. A physician, Sun Si Miao in *Qing Jin Yao Fang* (The Valuable Prescriptions) states "The mothers are not recommended to feed their child if they have diseases such as goiter, tumors, scrofula, asthma, scabies, tinea capitis, dementia, dysuria, deafness, epilepsy and mania."

How to help the nursing mother stay healthy?

In order to obtain and maintain optimal health it is recommended that the nursing mother follow the five flavor diet, stay calm and have a gentle temperament.

How to nurse

The below methods were recommended by ancient physicians:

Massage the breast before feeding in order to create smooth milk and to have better control over the flow of milk. Clean the nipple before and after feeding and expel stored milk. Don't nurse while a child is crying. Use a good nursing posture that won't obstruct the baby's nose while they are nursing or after they have finished and fall asleep. Have flexibility to adjust the nursing time and duration according to the child's needs. Once finished, hold them up with their head on the mother's shoulder and lightly tap their back to induce gas from their stomach, which helps prevent vomiting.

When and how to stop breastfeeding

Supplementary food such as porridge, rice gruel, noodles and eggs should be added gradually as breastfeeding is reduced. Breastfeeding frequency should be slowly reduced to a stop when the child is around one year old. If possible, weaning should not happen during the hottest part of summer or the coldest part of winter; it will make it more difficult for the child. Breastfeeding is strongly advocated and is very healthy for the baby. However, there are other ways to feed in cases where breastfeeding is not possible either due to insufficient milk production or other reasons. One may add cow's milk to the breast milk or formula, or they may feed completely with cow's milk or formula instead of breast milk. After one year of age the nature and quality of the child's food will have significant differences. With the gradual eruption of the deciduous teeth and increased chewing function, milk and liquids can no longer be staples for them. Therefore, the feeding should follow some fundamental guidelines.

A comprehensive blended diet

Sufficient staple food should be ensured as a foundation to the diet. All nutrition should meet the demands of their rapid growth and development. The diet includes five categories of food which include energy, structure, regulation, transport medium and detoxification. The seven nutritional categories are protein, fat, carbohydrates, water, vitamins, fiber and minerals. The diet should be reasonably arranged in terms of portion size and variety according to certain ratios: 10-15% protein, 25-30% fat, 50-60% carbohydrates. A variety of foods will complement the protein intake in order to maximize nutritional utilization. The following table can be used as a reference for the child's diet.

The daily need of food types and quantity for 1 to 3 year-old in grams

Rice or Wheat	Fat	Veggies & Fruit	Bean Products	Egg	Fish	Cow Milk	Sugar
150	25	100-150	50-100	50	50-100	250	10

Soft, Minced and Shredded Foods

A child has 20 teeth until two and a half years old. Babies and young children should be fed with relatively soft, minced and shredded food. This is more conducive to the child's digestion and absorption. One should avoid feeding greasy and irritating foods.

Feeding schedule

A child has to be fed regularly, on time and amounts must be controlled. They should not become excessively hungry or full. The Jing Yue Encyclopedia states: "The child who is biased with food suffers easily. It is said that cool tastes the comfort the child's mouth eventually leads them to illness."

Increase the baby's appetite with a pleasant environment

Parents also have to pay attention by creating a pleasant environment in which to enjoy meals. Teach them to be in a good mood while eating and to behave properly during meal time. For example, the parents should not force their children to take meals. Cook meals that have attractive colors, smells and tastes. Train the babies to feed themselves at about one year old. With patience, encouragement and education of the parents, the children will develop a robust appetite.

Highlights of Care

Pediatric care should take the following points according to the different ages of implementation:

- "If parents want their babies to be healthy, let them be slightly hungry and a little bit chilled" (Roots of Disease in Children, 1251). This is the experience of the ancient physicians who, according to the features of Pure Yang, Young Yin and Young Yang was a drawback of feeding if kids were kept too warm or fed too much. This means that a child's diet should be focused on regularity and moderation. They should be dressed appropriately for the weather with care taken not over or under dress them.
- It may damage the spleen if children are fed irregularly or overfed, and in turn, this can lead to damage of other zang fu organs. Dressing them too warm may aggravate Pure Yang and cause over sweating, resulting in a cold. Particular attention should be paid in not covering an infant's head too much.

This will hinder yang steaming from the body. A physician, Chen Wen Zhong in the Song Dynasty (960-1276) said in his *Ten Secrets of Nursing* "One of the most important factors is that the infant's head should be kept cool."

- Infants should be dressed in used cloth that will not irritate their skin or cause them to become too warm. Ancient physicians emphasized that "infants should be dressed in used cloth, not new cotton." New silk is not as good as used clothes and do not dress children in fur. In addition, it is better if children's clothes are made from cotton rather than silk. They recommended avoiding clothing that was too small or too tight. Parents should use more or less clothes based on the weather. The ancients also advocated parents to train their children to wear less clothing in general. The best time to train them in wearing less clothing is in the fall.

- Focus on establishing good sleeping and eating habits. Parents should try to create a good living environment that is appropriate for the children's age. The children's amount of rest and nutrition should be consistent with their changing needs as they grow. Children should be given adequate time for sleep, which is essential to their proper development. Training to create a healthy and regular sleep schedule should begin in early childhood. Follow these general guidelines: Newborns sleep about 20 hours a day. 6 months old sleep about 16 hours a day. 1 year olds sleep about 14 hours a day. 3 yearsolds sleep about 12 hours day.7 year olds need about 10 hours a day. 12~18 year olds need 9 hours a day.

- Warm sunshine and fresh air are important in the growth and development of children. General Treatise on the Causes and Symptoms of Diseases 616 CE suggests: "When the weather is warm and there is no wind, mother should hold her baby and play with him under the sunshine. Playing under the sun generates qi, blood, muscles and skin and will increase their ability to resist wind and cold. If they habitually wear too many layers of clothes and avoid being out in the sun, they will become weak like grasses without the sun and will be easily sick." Appropriate exposure to sunlight will strengthen the constitution of the child and decrease the incidence of diseases such as rickets and of the respiratory system.

- Vaccination can provide immunity to certain pathogens and is a key measure in the prevention of childhood infectious diseases. It should be noted on a schedule to complete a variety of vaccinations and establish the child's vaccination files.
- Correctly and carefully use herbs. Prescribed herbs in pediatrics have to be correct and prudent. Children are quickly responsive and sensitive to this therapy due to their clear, agile and effective zang qi. If they take the medication slightly incorrectly, it will not only be ineffective in the treatment of the illness, but will also affect the balance of yin and yang resulting in illness.

Characteristics in the Pediatric Clinic

Although the four diagnostics of pediatrics and the contents of TCM diagnostics are the same, differences exist between TCM diagnostics and pediatric clinical practice since children and adults differ morphologically, physiologically and pathologically. Therefore, pediatricians should understand the characteristics of pediatric diagnostic methods and grasp the main contents of the diagnostic characteristics of pediatrics.

Diagnostic characteristics

Pediatricians endeavor to use all four diagnostic methods. The methods of observation, auscultation, olfaction, inquiry, and body palpation are unique characteristics that can't be replaced. Practitioners can't comprehensively and systemically understand diseases and make the correct diagnosis and differentiation until they organically combine all data collected. However, there are difficulties in pediatrics. First, babies and young children either can't speak or their language is not understandable, which causes difficultly for practitioners to get information through inquiry. Second, it is difficult to get the information from observation, auscultation and olfaction, and body palpation if crying affects voice, color of face, spirit and pulse during the visit. Ancient physicians state there are five difficulties in pediatrics. *Xi Er Yao Zheng Zhi Jue* (The Keys to Differentiation and Treatment of Children's Diseases) says: "Even the Yellow Emperor had trouble in treating children's illnesses, the first difficulty is that the pulse of the child is difficult to be felt since their pulse is feeble and they will cry when they are checked by physicians, the second one is that physicians have to depend on the child's outside manifestations of the child, and their bones haven't developed completely. Their physical body and voices are changing, their mood changes frequently. The third, babies can't speak or their language is not understandable, which causes practitioners difficultly when get information from inquiry. The fourth, zang and fu of children are delicate, subject to vacuity and repletion syndromes (Yi Xu Yi Shi) and subject to cold and heat syndrome (Yi Han Yi Re)". A physician, Zhang Jing Yue in his book, *Jing Yue Quan Shu* (Encyclopedia of Jinyue) says "Pediatrics was called the mute department in the ancient times since physicians couldn't understand what children said, and their diseases were difficult to diagnose and differentiate. Therefore, practitioners would complain that they would rather they treat ten men than one woman, and prefer to treat ten women than one child. This indicates how difficult it was for pediatricians to treat children's diseases. In my opinion, the main difficulty of pediatrics is in the differentiation of syndromes. Because children cannot talk or explain what they are feeling, pediatrics was jokingly referred to as treating mutes.

Although pediatricians have difficulty in using all diagnostic methods in practice, the change of weakness and excess of qi and blood, yin and yang are easily showed through their skin because of the child's thin skin. All disorders in the internal must show at the external. Therefore, observation is emphasized strongly among the diagnostics in pediatrics. A physician in his book *You Ke Tie Jin Jing* (Pediatric Iron Mirror) in the Qing dynasty states "In pediatrics diagnostics, observation is first and mainly used, followed by inquiry, then auscultation and olfaction." The content of pediatric observation is very abundant. Practitioners have to pay attention and use the skills of observation carefully in pediatrics.

Observing the index vein is a unique diagnostic tool

Inspecting the index vein is a special diagnostic method created by ancient physicians based on pediatric observation. It is is mainly used in pediatrics for children under three years old, which is used to compensate for inadequacies of taking the pulse of children under three years old.

Collecting different information from the four diagnostics for different ages of children

Children have special physiological and pathological conditions because they keep growing and developing at different rates. For example, pediatricians have to observe the navel of the newborn, look at the fontanels of the baby and observe their index finger vein when they are younger than 3 years old.

Appropriate combining of modern diagnostic methods

With time progressing and the development of science, medicine is also constantly developing. It greatly helps and benefits physicians practicing pediatrics. All of the new and modern diagnostic methods have become an important part in pediatrics.

Diagnostic Methods

Observation

Pediatricians primarily focus on observation, but it is not easy. During inspection, first observe the child overall. Look at the body in general, including nutrition, growth, spirit, and awareness, then purposely and orderly carry out the comprehensive and focused inspection according to their diseases. Thus, physicians can find the positive symptoms and signs for making a diagnosis. The contents of inspection in pediatrics are inspecting spirit and facial complexion, bodily form, orifices, skin rashes and eruptions, stool and urination, and the index vein.

Inspecting the Spirit (Vitality) and Facial Complexion

Broadly speaking, the spirit is the outward manifestation of a person's activities and lifestyle, including the vitality and dynamics of the body. The narrow sense of the human spirit is a thinking activity. The *Nei Jing* says: "Spirit is from the essence of foods", which means the spirit is based on the yin essence. Physicians can detect the functional states of zang and fu, the severity and prognosis of the diseases by inspecting the child's spirit and determine the sufficiency or weakness of essence. The following inspection can help determine whether the spirit is normal or lacking.

- brightness or dullness of eyes.
- clearness or unclear of consciousness.
- coherence or incoherence of movement.
- agility of reaction.

The manifestations of a normal spirit are a clear mind, bright eyes, flexible movement, and coherent responses. Otherwise, there is a lack of spirit. We must observe the skin color and luster. Inspecting color mainly means looking at the facial complexion. Children who are from different nationalities, endowments and other factors may have differing skin colors, such as a little white or slightly yellow, or a little black, but the normal facial complexion is always shiny and lustrous.

A pale facial complexion is related to the lung, which indicates cold and vacuity. If the complexion is pale, with goose bumps, it suggests an exterior wind-cold syndrome. If the complexion is pale with puffy eye lids and edema of the legs, this is yang vacuity of the spleen and kidney. If the complexion is accompanied by emaciation, this is qi and blood vacuity. A yellow facial complexion is related to the spleen, and indicates vacuity and dampness. A withered yellow color is qi and blood vacuity due to insufficiency of the spleen. A bright yellow color indicates damp-heat, which leads to jaundice manifested with yellow urination and yellow sclera. A red complexion that is related to the heart indicates a heat syndrome. A red facial complexion in the whole face, even in the ears means excessive heat syndrome. If the cheeks are redder than other parts of the face it is a vacuity heat syndrome. If only the cheeks are redder without being shiny, and it looks like make up, accompanied by cold extremities, this indicates exhaustion of yang caused by yang counter-flowing upward because yang is too weak to be kept at the root. Green-blue and purple is related to the liver and indicates the syndromes of wind, pain, blood stasis and convulsion. If the cheeks are green-blue, this indicates convulsion. If there is a green-blue complexion accompanied with crying, this indicates abdominal pain. If the vein at the root of the bridge of the nose between the two eyes, which is "Shan Gen" in Chinese, is visible and purple, this indicates that the liver is overacting on the spleen, or there is a wind-heat syndrome. If there are blue-purple lips, this suggests pneumonia due to obstruction of the lung qi. A green-blue complexion accompanied by chronic vomiting and diarrhea, suggests chronic convulsion. If there is a purple and black color all around the lips, this indicates severe depletion of the liver and kidney. Black complexion, the color of kidney, indicates cold, pain, body fluid retention, and poor prognosis. If there is a green and black complexion with severe abdominal pain, this suggests interior yin cold syndrome. If there is black around the lips without brightness, it indicates exhaustion of kidney. If the eye lids are black and puffy accompanied with edema, clear and profuse urination during the night, this suggests kidney vacuity. It is more significant if the indications of the five complexion diagnostics combine with the five areas of face. The five locations are related five zang, The forehead relates to the heart, the nose to the spleen, the left cheek to the liver, the right cheek to the lung, and the chin to the kidney.

Inspecting the bodily form and movement

Inspecting the bodily form includes the body, generally, and local parts. Understanding the general state of the body through observing the development and nutrition is important. If the child shows normal development, strong bones and muscles, shiny skin, lively attitude, this means the bodily form is strong; otherwise, the child is sick. Inspecting the local parts includes observing the skull and fontanels, neck, trunk, extremity, skin, hair, fingers and toes.

Inspecting the head, skull, fontanels and neck

Check the size of the skull and whether or not there is deformity of the head and skull. Look at the size of the fontanels and observe if they have closed early or late and if there are bulges or depressions around the fontanels. Observe if the neck is soft, hard, oblique, and normally active. Check if the neck veins are bulged.

Inspecting the trunk

This includes inspecting the shape of the thoracodorsal spine, abdomen, umbilical area and waist, the skin condition and muscle development.

Inspecting the extremities

Mainly inspect the shape of the limbs, skin, muscles and limbs.

Inspecting the skin

Pay attention to the skin color, status, appearance of rash etc. Be careful to note the condition of the skin in particular areas as they relate to associated zang organ correlations.

Inspecting the hair

Mainly look at the hair color and distribution of the hair, if it is thin or dense.

Inspecting the nails

Check the color and shapes of the nails.

Observing the orifices

The orifices refer to the senses of eyes, ears, nose, and mouth. The nine orifices externally show signs of the five zang. The tongue is the sprout of heart, the eyes are the orifice to the liver, the nose is the orifice to the lung, and the mouth is the orifice to the spleen. The ears, urethra and anus are the orifices to the kidney. *An Iron Mirror of Pediatrics* says: "There will be external manifestations, when the children suffer internally. The five zang are not viewed, but their orifices are seen absolutely." Physicians will certainly know the repletion and vacuity of the zang fu organs, if the colors of the orifices and facial complexions match. Inspecting the orifices can detect the changes of cold, heat, repletion and vacuity of the corresponding zang fu. Therefore, it is a very important diagnostic tool in pediatrics.

Inspecting the eyes

Pay attention to the spirit, shape, color and movement of the eyes, and combine these observations with the related locations in the eyes that correspond to the internal zang fu. The heart shows at the canthus, the spleen at the eye lids, lungs at the sclera, the liver at the iris, and the kidneys at the pupil. If the eyes are red, this indicates yang repletion syndrome. Congestion of the whole eye with swelling, pain and excessive secretions indicates heat in the liver. Yellow sclera that is shiny suggests damp-heat. Green sclera indicates excessive wind. Contracted pupils suggest the vacuity of liver and kidney. Watering eyes indicate an early sign of measles. Sunken eyes indicate vacuity of body fluid. Staring eyes indicates infantile convulsions. Pale eyelids indicate blood vacuity.

Inspecting the nose

Mainly inspect the form, color, and discharge of the nose. Green-blue nose indicates chronic pain. Clear discharge is wind cold, and turbid discharge is wind heat. Shortness of breath with nares flaring suggests pneumonia. If there is a yellow and sticky discharge that has an odor, this indicates rhinorrhea. if the nose is bleeding, this indicates lung heat with Yin vacuity. Redness inside of the nose indicates excessive heat in the lungs.

Inspecting the mouth

This includes looking at the lips, teeth, gums, throat, cheeks, jaw and tongue. Inspecting the lips involves mainly looking at the color, moisture level, and whether there is ulceration. Inspecting the teeth involves looking at the number of primary or permanent teeth, and determining whether it matches their age or not. Also observe the color and shape of the teeth. Inspecting the gums involves looking at the color and condition of the gums. Observing the throat in clinical pediatrics is very important and is especially helpful in diagnosing the disorders of the lung and spleen. Inspection of the throat is to mainly observe whether tonsils are red, swollen, or even ulcerative or purulent. Proper visibility of the throat requires that the tongue be pressed by a depressor; it might be better to perform this examination after collecting all of the child's information.

Before the doctor inspects the throat, the parents should hold the child's hand. Next, the doctor should hold the depressor in one hand while the other hand positions the child's head to a light source. The doctor should quickly and lightly press the depressor to the root of the tongue and observe the throat. Inspecting the cheek and jaw, mainly consists of observing the shape and color inside the cheek. Inspecting the tongue is one of the most important components of pediatrics. The contents of observing the tongue in pediatrics are similar to the contents of the tongue in internal medicine, but practitioners should note that a normal tongue varies with age. For example, the normal tongue of a newborn is red and without coating, while the normal tongue of an infant is pink tongue and with a white coating.

Inspecting the ears

Look at the shape, the color, and if there is secretion in ears or lymph nodes behind the ears.

Inspecting the anus and urethra

Look at the shape and the color of the anus and urethra. If the scrotum of a boy is tight with a purplish color, this indicates the boy is healthy. On the other hand, if it is slacken with a pale color, it suggests the boy is sick. If girls frequently get urinary tract infections that could be due to anatomical abnormalities of the urethra.

Distinguishing rashes and macula

Rashes and macula are common manifestations in pediatrics, and are the signs of general diseases that reflect in the body surface. It is helpful for pediatricians to not only make a diagnosis, but also indicates the severity and progression of diseases based on distinguishing the different shapes, distribution, color, appearance and disappearance of the rashes and macula. The common warm diseases, such as measles, rubella, Dan Sha (Scalate Fever), Nai Ma (Exanthema Subitum) have their own difference (Please refer to Infectious Diseases).

Inspecting the stool and urine

Inspect the frequency, volume, color, smell and shape of the stool. The feces of healthy infants are different because of their different diet. The feces of infants who are breastfed are 2 or 3 times per day, loose, yellow, few milk clots, and have a sour smell. The feces of infants who are fed cow milk are slightly dry, once per day, easy to constipation, and pale yellow. There are more milk clots in the feces, and the odor is stronger. After the normal feces of the infant are fully understood, the abnormal stools can be distinguished.

Inspecting the index vein

Mainly inspect the location and clinical indications of the index vein. The location of the index finger vein refers to the exposed vein on the palmar aspect of the index finger, which is a branch of the lung meridian of hand Taiyin. It belongs to the category of taking the Cunkou pulse in diagnosis. It is used to diagnose diseases for infants younger than three years old instead of standard pulse-taking. The index finger vein is divided into three passes or bars. From the cross striation of the metacarpo-phalangeal joint to that of the second phalanx is the wind pass. From the cross striation of the second phalanx to that of the third phalanx, is the qi pass. From the cross of striation of the third phalanx to the pit of the index finger, is the life-pass.

The method of inspecting the index vein

First, the parents should have their infant face the light. Next, while holding the infant's index finger with the left hand, the physician should put his right thumb on the infant's index vein, then gently and continually push forward from the life pass to the qi pass and to the wind pass, and repeat several times.

The indications of inspecting index vein

The normal index vein is light red and is indistinct within the wind pass. It is not invisible but not obvious either. A floating or deep index vein distinguishes the exterior syndrome from interior syndrome: If the index vein is obviously visible, it is a floating index vein, which indicates the infant has an exterior syndrome. If it is obscure, it suggests an interior syndrome. A pale red or purple index vein differentiates cold and heat syndromes. If the index vein is pale red, it means cold syndrome. If it is purple, it is due to a heat syndrome. If it is floating and pale red, it is exterior wind-cold syndrome. A deep, pale red color indicates an interior cold syndrome. A floating and purple index vein indicates an exterior wind-heat while a deep and purple vein indicates interior heat. Smooth or stagnation discerns vacuity or repletion. Smooth indicates that the blood flow in the index vein is smooth and it recovers quicker than normal after being pushed, this indicates vacuity. Stagnation means the blood flow in the index vein is sluggish and it recovers slower than normal, this indicates a repletion syndrome. The three passes predict the severity of the disease. The index vein in the wind pass means the child is not sick or only mildly sick. If it is in the qi pass, this indicates the illness is severe. If it is in the life pass, this is even more severe. "Tou Guan She Jia" refers to the index vein passing from the wind pass to the qi pass, life pass the tip of the nail, this phenomenon suggests the illness is critical.

There is certain clinical importance in inspecting the index vein, but practitioners have to "She Wen Cong Zheng" (Diagnose depending on the differentiation syndromes and abandoning the index vein) if the indication of index vein doesn't match the syndrome.

Listening and smelling

Listening is used to differentiate the diseases according to the sound of the child's crying, language, coughing, breathing and other noises that can be heard. Crying is the language of an infant and is a common expression of physical discomfort. It is normal for healthy children to cry loudly with tears several times a day. The following situations may also cause crying, such as hunger, a wet diaper, tight clothing and other improper care. If an infant cries sharply, suddenly, expresses panic, or cries with moaning, practitioners need to observe and check very carefully.

In addition to listening with the ears, the stethoscope can be used to check the the speed, depth, or rhythm of breathing and if there are rales of the lungs. Fine and moist rales in the lungs suggests pneumonia.

Smelling involves inspecting the odor of the breath, secretions and excretions. Many diseases can a have special smell that can help with the diagnosis. For example, vomiting with an odor that is milky and rotten sour indicates food stagnation. Foul breath indicates heat accumulation in the stomach. Purulent nasal discharge with a fishy odor indicates a case of naso-sinusitis.

These are the following characteristics in pediatric inquiry:

The person you are inquiring is not the patient and therefore may not offer a complete and fully reliable account. In addition to the inquiry, the contents of pediatrics are similar to the contents of TCM diagnostics. The followings are carefully asked:

- age of the child in months or days
- natural birth or cesarean
- feeding methods
- developmental history
- vaccination history

Note the art of interrogation and attitudes. While obtaining the information, practitioners should try to use words and sentences that are familiar to children, and try to get the cooperation of both the parents and children.

Body palpation

This includes pulse taking and body palpation. These are the following characteristics in pediatric pulse taking.

- For children under 3 years old, it is generally not necessary to take the pulse. Instead, inspect the index vein. Practitioners may use "one finger taking Cunkou pulse method" or one finger taking the Cun, Guan, Chi gates of pulse for elder than 3 years old.
- The rates of a normal pulse is different among the ages, the younger the age, the faster the pulse rate (see the table below).
- It is not necessary for pediatricians to distinguish among the 28 kinds of pulse in children, but they have to consider the 6 types of pulses including floating, deep, slow, rapid, strong and weak pulses. These help to guide diagnosis between the exterior or interior, cold or heat, repletion or vacuity.
- The indications of pulse taking in different ages are different.

The rates of pulse and respiration in different ages:

Ages	Breath (times/minute)	Pulse (times/minute)	breath:pulse
newborn	40~45	120~140	1:3
<1year	30~40	110~130	1:3~4
2~3years	25~30	100~120	1:3~4
4~7years	20~25	80~100	1:4
8~14years	18~20	70~90	1:4

Body palpation for children is noted in the followings:

- Palpate the head and occipital skull of the baby, to understand if fontanels are closed or not, protruding or sunken, or if the skull is soft like a table tennis ball.

- It is easier to palpate the child's abdomen when the child is quiet, or while the infant is breast feeding.
- It is normal if the liver's edge extends past the ribs 1-2cm, but it should not be clear on palpation after 7 years old.

Summary of Differentiation

Characteristics of differentiation

This section emphasizes that the differentiation of syndromes should be timely and accurate. Children have the physiological characteristics of Pure Yang, Young Yin and Young Yang and the pathological characteristics that are subject to vacuity and repletion syndromes and are subject to cold and heat syndromes. Since the syndromes of children may change several times in a day, practitioners have to act in a timely manner and accurately differentiate the syndromes of children's diseases in order to apply appropriate therapy. To distinguish the chief syndrome and accompanying syndrome The syndromes of children are mostly mixed repletion with vacuity and heat with cold. Practitioners have to distinguish the chief syndrome from the mixed syndrome, and then determine the therapy mainly for the chief syndrome and partially for accompanying symptoms. For example, the phlegm-heat accumulating the lung may be the chief syndrome of pediatric pneumonia, and it is commonly accompanied by heart qi vacuity. The main therapy is clearing heat, expelling phlegm, and opening the lung qi. The adjuvant therapy is supplementing heart qi. When the child has obvious heart qi vacuity or even exhaustion of heart yang, the main therapy should be changed to restoring the yang, strongly supplementing source qi, and rescuing the qi from collapse. When creating a diagnosis, it is important to prioritize and address all identified patterns. For example, pneumonia and acute glomerulonephritis, both of which may cause the exhaustion of heart Yang syndrome. However, they have different basic pathologies. Pediatric pneumonia is due to phlegm-heat accumulating in the lung, while acute glomerulonephritis is due to damp-heat accumulating in the triple burner, waterway congestion and water accumulating in the lung and attacking the heart. There may be more difficulty in curing the disease if practitioners simply treat the exhaustion of heart yang for the two diseases.

Summary of Therapy

The treatment is the final key for clinical success. The correct and effective therapy is based on the guidance of the principles of TCM and pediatric characteristics. I must emphasize that the treatment should be timely, accurate and cautious. Diseases occur rapidly and change rapidly in children. Their illnesses can be cured or worsened in a moment, so it is important to grasp the pathology and treat it in time. The response to therapy in children is sensitive. This is because children's yang qi is clear, agile and effective. The treatment is closely related to the advance or retreat of diseases, therefore, the treatment used for children must be very cautious, especially for newborns and infants.

Note the choice and dosage of herbs

The formulas or herbs should be selected and used appropriately according to physical characteristics of children. All of the formulas or herbs that are strong toxic, acrid, hot, cold, and heavy in weight or purge are cautiously used for children. When prescribing these group formulas or herbs, practitioners should follow the principle "when the disease is removed by half, the medicine should be ceased."

Try to use the appropriate pharmaceutical preparation. It is inconvenient for children to take herbal decoctions. Also, the slow effect of decoction are often unsuitable for treating acute and critical conditions. Practitioners have to make use of the indications of pharmaceutical preparations for different diseases of children.

The methods of decoction

Herbal decoction is the most frequently used form in pediatrics. The following table shows suggested dosage based on age.

The dosage of herb and volume of decoction in different ages:

Ages	Dosage of herb (?/adult)	Volume of decoction(ml)
<1year	1/6~1/4	30~50
1~3years	1/3~1/2	50~100
4~7years	1/2~2/3	100~150
8~14years	2/3~1/1	150~200

Commonly used methods of treatment in pediatrics

Release the exterior

This is used for the exterior syndrome and Wei (defensive) syndrome, which includes the methods that release the exterior wind-cold with acrid warm herbs, release the exterior wind-heat with acrid cold herbs and release the exterior and summer heat. Releasing the exterior with acrid cold herbs is more commonly used in pediatrics. Children who have the exterior or Wei level syndromes easily have complications, such as cough and wheezing due to phlegm, vomiting and diarrhea due to food stagnation, or convulsion due to high fever. Therefore, the method of releasing the exterior is often used with the method of opening lung qi and resolving phlegm, digesting food stagnation, calming wind and stopping convulsion. The common formulas are Sang Ju Yin (Mulberry and Chrysanthemum Decoction) and Yin Qiao San (Honeysuckle and Forsythia Powder). The points are Du14 (Ga Zhui), LI11 (Qu Chi), LI4 (He Gu).

Stop cough and arrest asthma

"Cough may be caused by all disorders of the five zang and six fu, not only by disorder of the lung, but it always relates to the lung." The location of the cough is in the lung, and is caused by the lung failing to ascend and descend. The basic therapy of stopping cough and arresting asthma is descending and ascending the lung qi, which acts in concert with clearing the lung, warming the lung, drying damp and eliminating phlegm. There are representative formulas, such as Ma Xing Shi Gan Tang (Ephedra, Apricot, Licorice and Gypsum Decoction), Xiao Qing Long Tang (Minor Blue Green Dragon Decoction), Liu An Jian (Six-Serenity Decoction), Qing Qi Hua Tan Wan (Clear the Qi and Transform Phlegm Pill).

Clear heat and relieve toxicity

Children mostly suffer from heat syndromes and it turns into fire and toxicity, because their constitutions belong to Pure Yang. This method includes the method of using acrid and cold, bitter and cold, salty and cold, bitter and purging herbs. The heat and toxins can be in a lot of different locations, such as the Wei, Qi, Ying and Blood levels, in the zang fu organs, the exterior, the interior, and in the half exterior and half interior. The representative formulas are Yin Qiao San (Honeysuckle and Forsythia Powder), Bai Hu Tang (White Tiger Decoction), Qing Ying Tang (Clear the nutritive level decoction), Xie Bai San (Purging White Powder), Huang Lian Jie Du Tang (Coptis Detoxicating Decoction), Qing Wen Bai Du Yin (Clear Eepidemics and Overcome Toxin Decoction), and so on. This group's formulas can be overused for children for they are both Pure Yang and Young Yang. The child's yang might be injured if these are overused.

Transform the spleen and increase appetite

The pediatric spleen is commonly insufficient, and the stomach is small and tender and thus cannot contain a large amount of food. Therefore, children easily suffer spleen and stomach disorders. There are therapeutic methods for increasing appetite, including supplementing the spleen's function of transportation and transformation, and helping the stomach receive food. The representative formulas are Si Shi Wan (Increasing appetite Pill), Yi Wei Tang (Benefit the Stomach Decoction), Qi Wei Bai Zhu San (Seven- Ingredient powder with Atractylodes Macrocephala), Shen Ling Bai Zhu San (Ginsen, Poria, and Atractylodes Macrocephala Powerder), Li Zhong Tang (Regulate the Middle Pill). The Tuina and food therapy are also widely used for this method.

Aid digestion and purge stagnation

If children are improperly fed, the transportation and transformation of the spleen and stomach will easily be impaired, which could lead to milk or food stagnation and is manifested by fever, abdominal pain, vomiting, diarrhea and malnutrition. The goals of this therapy use a combination of herbs that reduce food stagnation and regulate qi. The representative formulas are Bao He Wan (Preserve Harmony Pill), Xia Ru Wan (Reduce Milk Stagnation Pill), and Zhi Shi Dao Zhi (Immature Bitter Orange Pill to Guide out Stagnation). The herbs that reduce food stagnation are used selectively, such as Shan Zha (Fructus Crataegi), Chao Mai Ya (Fried Fructus Hordei Vulgaris germinantus), Chao Gu Ya (Fructus Oryzae Sativae Germinantus), and Ji Nei Jin (Endothelium Cornei Gigeriae Galli) according to the type of food stagnation.

Calm the spirit and open the orifices

The diseases that children mostly suffer from belong to heat syndromes, which may eventually stir up wind, and cause convulsion. Another cause of convulsion could be fluid that is burned by heat and transformed into phlegm that heats the heart orifice. Therefore, this therapy is usually used for the acute and febrile diseases in children. The representatives are An Gong Niu Huang Wan (Calm the Palace Pill with Cattle Gallstone), Zhi Bao Dan (Greatest Treasure Special Pill), Zi Xue Dan (Purple Snow Special Pill), Ling Jiao Gou Teng Tang (Antelope Horn and Uncaria Decoction). There are modern herbal preparations in recent years, such as intravenous herbal agent, Qing Kai Ling (Clear and Open the Spirit of Intravenous).

Invigorate the blood stasis

This is used mostly for chronic illness and difficult diseases, such as pediatric pneumonia, asthma, nephritic syndromes, and purpura. The representatives are Dan Hong Yin (Salvia and Safflower Decoction), Tao Hong Si Wu Tang (Four-Substance Decoction with Safflower and Peach), Xue Fu Zhu Yu Tang (Drive Out Stasis in the Mansion of Blood Decoction).

Nourish Yin and supplement qi

Children easily get heat syndromes when they get sick. The constitution of children is Pure Yang; however, they also easily have the syndrome of qi and yin vacuity because their constitution is made of Young Yin and Young Yang. Therefore, this therapy is more widely used in the late stages of warm febrile diseases. The representatives are Sha Shen Mai Dong Tang (Glehnia and Ophiopoponis Decoction), Yi Wei Tang (Benefit the Stomach Decoction), and Sheng Mai San (Generate the Pulse Powder).

Rescue devastated yang

These are used to restore exhausted yang. The representatives are Shen Fu Tang(Ginseng and Prepared Aconite Decoction) and Si Ni Tang(Frigid Extremities Decoction).

External therapy

External therapy is the application of medicinals to areas such as the skin, orifices, and acupuncture points. Advantages of this therapy include increased safety, easier use, wide indications and the ability to reach the affected area directly. Hence, external therapy is an important supplement to internal therapy.

Steaming and washing therapy

The affected part of the body is soaked, steamed or washed by a warm herbal decoction. This has the function of expelling cold and stopping pain and itching, and promoting rashes. Depending on the medicinal functions, steaming and washing therapy can promote the circulation of qi and blood, and open the skin and muscles. It is mostly used for rashes, skin diseases and swelling and pain in local areas. For example, the decoction for washing with the herbs, such as Cang Er Zi(Fructus Xanthi)), Bai Ji Li (Fructus Tribuli Terrestris), Bai Xian Pi (Cortex Dictammi Dasycarpi), She Chuang Zi (Fructus Cnidii Monnier)), and Chan Tui (Periostracum Cicadae) are effective for urticaria.

Topical therapy

Pounded medicinals mixed with various liquids can be applied to certain parts of the body for treating local disorders. This therapy has the functions of regulating yin and yang, zang-fu, qi and blood. The indications for its use include local illness, and internal disorders, such as mumps, enuresis, diarrhea, and asthma. Its effectiveness is amplified when combined with other therapies.

Smearing therapy

The herbal decoction, medicated wine, and ointment are applied onto certain parts of the body surface. These are used most commonly in traumatic injury and skin disorders. For example, Zi Cao oil is used for treating reddish rashes on the buttock.

Hot compress therapy

This is the external application of a hot medicated pad over the affected area or acupoint. It is used for eliminating blood stasis, accelerating the reduction in swelling, promoting blood circulation and relieving pain.

Inhalation therapy

This is effective only when the inhaled herbal particles reach the throat and lungs, where they can deliver their effects. This medication inhalation is done with the help of an inhaler device. It is used for cough, pneumonia, and asthma. The common herbs are Zhu L i(Dried Bamboo Sap) and Yu Xing Cao (houttuynia cordata).

Other therapies

Tuina

It is also known as massage. Pediatric massage is unique and has a long history. It is widely used for disorders of the spleen, stomach, lung, five sense organs, traumatology, and the nervous system. Tuina also can promote the growth and development of children. There are different indications of various kinds of manipulations of Tuina. The pinching spine technique is effective for food stagnation, while the pushing and rolling technique is used for constipation and diarrhea.

Acupuncture

Acupuncture manipulation techniques for children are the same as that of an adult, but it is better for children when they are needled quickly, superficially, and without needle retention. The common indications for acupuncture are disorders of the spleen and stomach, enuresis, trauma, and refractory syndromes of pediatrics. Practitioners have to pay special attention when burning moxa on children.

Food therapy

Diet therapy should be modified according to the differentiation of syndromes. For example, Xing Li Yin (almond and pearl drink) is good for pneumonia due to wind-heat. Lu Gen Yu Xing Cao Dong Gua Yin (Reed Fishy Grass Winter Melon Drink) is for pneumonia due to phlegm heat. Generally, greasy, spicy, and very sweet food should be limited or avoided.

Diseases of the newborn infant

The diseases that occur during the newborn phase of life have the following features:

- There is a high incidence of mortality due to insufficiency of qi and blood
- The diseases that newborn infants suffer from are quite different than those of children of other ages.
- The common causes of newborn infant diseases are congenital malformations, birth trauma, asphyxia, infection, premature birth and intrauterine growth retardation.
- Diseases of newborns often lack the typical clinical manifestations. For example, neonatal pneumonia and asthma may only present with vomiting of foamy fluid and purple lips, but no fever.

The causes of newborn diseases include those that are congenital and those that are acquired. Congenital causes are insufficiency of innate endowment such as neonatal weakness, neonatal heat and cold. Acquired causes are dystocia, improper omphalotomy or improper nursing and care. The incidence of neonatal diseases can be decreased by promoting fetal care and nursing. The history of the pregnancy and birth should be inquired in detail and it would probably be most effective by combining modern diagnostic techniques and TCM's diagnostic methods.

Neonatal Jaundice (Tai Huang 胎黄)

Neonatal jaundice manifests with yellowish skin, yellow sclera and yellow urine in the newborn. It is known as neonatal jaundice because of its occurrence in this phase of life. It includes physiological and pathological features. This section focuses on the treatment of neonatal jaundice.

Neonatal jaundice was first identified in the Sui Dynasty (581-618 A.D). In the book titled *Zhu Bing Yuan Hou Lun, Xiao Er Za Bing Hou,* (General Treatise on the Causes and Symptoms of Diseases,) 610, said "because the fetus lives in the uterus, if the pregnant woman has heat in her zang organs, this can steam the fetus causing neonatal jaundice." In the *Zheng Zhi Zhun Chun* (Standard for Diagnosis and Treatment) 1602, it states that neonatal jaundice is caused by "pregnant women who have dampness and heat that transfer to the fetus". From then on physicians have known that neonatal jaundice is not only related to congenital mechanisms, but also to the delivery process and acquired infections.

Etiology and Pathology

Neonatal jaundice is mainly caused by damp-heat accumulating in the woman during pregnancy and then transferring to the fetus, or the newborn is exposed to dampness and heat after birth.

Patterns

Damp-heat accumulation

After the damp-heat invades the newborn, it accumulates in the spleen and stomach, steaming the liver and gallbladder. The bile is forced out to the skin and eyes showing the signs of neonatal jaundice. Yang jaundice is the type caused by damp-heat steaming the liver and gall bladder. When there are critical symptoms such as convulsions and loss of consciousness, the mechanism is damp-heat transforming into fire with fire invading the Jueyin.

Damp-Cold accumulation

Cold-damp accumulation is considered a congenital vacuity. The weakness of the spleen, specifically spleen yang leads to dampness invading the spleen, blocking spleen yang, then disrupting the coursing and discharge function of the liver. Therefore, jaundice occurs. Yin jaundice is the type caused by damp-cold accumulation weakening the spleen yang. This manifests with a yellow, dull complexion and fatigue.

Jaundice due to blood stagnation

Congenital insufficiency with dampness in the spleen can lead to stasis of qi and blood. Blood stasis obstructs the meridians resulting in the dysfunction of soothing the liver and bile excretion from the gall bladder. Therefore, jaundice occurs.

Summary

Neonatal jaundice is related to congenital insufficiency and the invasion of dampness or damp-heat. The pathogenesis is dampness or damp heat accumulating in the spleen and stomach, failure in soothing of the liver, and bile moving out to the skin. The location of the disorder is mainly at the spleen, stomach, liver and gall bladder.

Diagnosis

Diagnostic guidelines

Any of the following features characterizes pathological jaundice:

- Clinical jaundice appearing in the first 24 hours or 2 to 3 weeks after birth, or reoccurring once initially relieved.
- More severe jaundice will show bilirubin direct more than 34 umol/l (2.0 mg/dL). Increases in the level of total

bilirubin by more than 8.5 umol/l (0.5 mg/dL) per hour. Total bilirubin more than 331.5 umol/l (19.5 mg/dL).
- Accompanying symptoms include fatigue, sleepiness or restlessness, poor appetite.

Diagnostic Notes

- Any history of maternal infection, medications, family history of hepatitis and birth of the newborn should be noted.
- The yellowish skin, sclera and urination should be observed carefully, particularly the sclera.
- The liver and spleen should be palpated carefully, while masses or abdominal fullness should be noted
- The pathological neonatal jaundice results from many mechanisms, such as hemolytic disease of the newborn, neonatal hepatitis syndrome, occlusion of neonatal biliary tract and neonatal sepsis. These must be differentiated not only depending on the history, manifestation and signs, but laboratory findings. For example, blood type of both the mother and infant is identified, blood serum bilirubin, liver function, ultrasound imaging of liver and gallbladder.

Differential Diagnosis

Physiological Neonatal Jaundice

The newborn will begin to show signs of jaundice 2 to 3 days after birth and the signs will disappear in 10 to 14 days. In a premature infant jaundice may last up to 3 or 4 weeks. The appetite will be normal, sleep will be normal and no other manifestations will appear.

Differentiation of Syndromes

Keys to differentiation

Differentiate between physiological and pathological neonatal jaundice Assess the infant's appearance, the duration of the jaundice, the severity of the jaundice and accompanying symptoms.

Differentiate between patterns due to cold, heat or blood stasis

If there is a bright yellowness with a red tongue, yellow tongue coating and a short history this is a damp-heat pattern. If there is a dull yellowness with a pale tongue, a white and greasy tongue coating and a longer history, this is a damp-cold pattern. If the jaundice continues to get worse with palpation of a hard mass in the abdomen, a purple tongue, a choppy pulse, this pattern is due to blood stasis.

Therapeutic Principle

Physiological jaundice will usually resolve on its own without treatment. The general treatment principle for pathological dampness is to drain damp to relieve jaundice.

Pattern Differentiation

Damp-heat accumulation

Manifestations: Bright yellow sclera and skin, fatigue, anxiety and crying, no appetite, deep yellow and scanty urine, red tongue with purple color and stagnated index vein.

Treatment Principle clear heat, drain dampness and resolve jaundice.

Formula: Yin Chen Hao Tang (Artemisia Yinchenhao decoction)

Yin Chen Hao (Herba Artemisiae Yinchenhao) clears heat, drains dampness and resolve jaundice. Zhi Zi (Fructus Gardeniae Jasminoidis) clears heat and dampness in three Jiao. Da Huang (Radix et Rhizoma Rhei) clears heat, drains fire and removes blood stasis. If there is no constipation, remove Da Huang. If there is vomiting, add Chen Pi (Pericarpium Citri Reticulatae), Zhu Ru (Phyllostachys Nigra), Ban Xia (Pinellia Ternatae) to eliminate phlegm and stop vomiting. If the patient has severe scanty and yellow urine, add Ze Xie (Alisma Plantago-aquatica) and Che Qian Cao (Herba Plantaginis) to drain dampness. If there is abdominal fullness add Hou Po (Cotex Magnoliae Officinalis), Zhi Shi (Fructus Immaturus Citri Aurantii) to regulate qi.

Damp-cold accumulation

Manifestations: Dull yellow sclera and skin, chronic fatigue, cold extremities, poor appetite, loose and clay-colored stool. Pale tongue with white greasy coating, pale index vein.

Treatment Principle Warm the middle, drain dampness and resolve jaundice.

Formula: Yin Chen Li Zhong Tang (Artemisia Yin Chen Hao Rectify the Middle Decoction)

Yin Chen Hao (Herba Artemisiae Yinchenhao) drains dampness and resolve jaundice. Gan Jiang (Rhizoma Zinggiberis Officinalis) warms and expels cold. Dang Shen (Radix Codonopsitis Pilosulae), Bai Zhu (Rhizoma Atractylodis), Fu Ling (Sclerotium Poria Cocos), Gan Cao (Radix Glycyrrhizae) supplement the spleen and drain dampness. Fu Zi (Radix Aconiti Lateralis Praeparata) and Gui Zhi (Ramulus Cinnamomi Cassiae) can be added for severely cold extremities. If there is abdominal mass due to blood stasis, add Dang Gui (Radix Angelicae Sinensis), Dan Shen (Radix Salviae Miltiorrhizae), E Zhu (Rhizoma Curcumae) and San Leng (Rhizoma Sparganii) to remove blood stasis. This syndrome is chronic and has a long history of illness. Practitioners should not only maintain the strategy and formulas, but also combine TCM and Western medicine.

Jaundice due to blood stasis

Manifestations: Jaundice becomes worse and worse, bright yellow skin at the beginning becoming a purplish yellow in the later stages, abdominal distention, lumpiness under right rib-side, low energy, and clay-colored stool. Purple tongue, stagnated and purple index vein.

Treatment Principle Remove blood stasis, soothe liver and resolve jaundice.

Formula: Xue Fu Zhu Yu Tang (Drive out Stasis in the Mansion of Blood Stasis Decoction).

Tao Ren (Semen Persicae), Hong Hua (Flos Carthami Tinctorii), Dang Gui (Radix Angelicae Sinensis), Chuang Xiong (Radix Ligustici Chuanxiong), Chi Shao (Radix Paeoniae Rubra), Niu Xi (Radix Achyranthis Bidentatae) for removing blood stasis. Chai Hu (Radix Bupleuri), Zhi Ke (Fructus Aurantii) for regulating liver Qi. Yin Chen Hao (Herba Artemisiae Yinchenhao) is often added in this formulas for resolve jaundice. If severe loose stool, Dang Shen (Radix Codonopsitis Pilosulae), Bai Zhu (Rhizoma Atractylodis), Fu Ling (Sclerotium Poria Cocos) are added for supplementing spleen and draining dampness.

Other Therapy

- Herbal enema- Yin Chen Hao (Herba Artemisiae Yinchenhao) 20g, Zhi Zi (Fructus Gardeniae Jasminoidis)10g and Da Huang (Radix et Rhizoma Rhei)2g, decoct all of them to about 100cc, do the enema 1-2x/day. This is used for neonatal jaundice due to damp heat.
- External Wash- Decoct Huang Bai (Cotex Phellodendri) 30g, and wash the infant 1-2 times/day. This is used for neonatal jaundice due to damp-heat.

Prevention and care

- The mother's diet during pregnancy and lactation, should be light, relatively bland and nutritious. She should avoid alcohol and greasy, cold and spicy foods.
- Pregnant women who previously delivered hemolytic babies may take the following herbs to prevent neonatal jaundice. The herbs are Yin Chen Hao (Herba Artemisiae Yinchenhao), Huang Qin (Radix Scutellariae Baicalensis), Bai Zhu (Rhizoma Atractylodis), Fu Ling (Sclerotium Poria Cocos), Dang Gui (Radix Angelicae Sinensis), Bai Shao (Radix Paeoniae Lactiflorae), Qi Zi (Fructus Lycii), Yi Mu Cao (Herba Leonuri Heterophylli).

Sclerema Neonatorum
(Xin Sheng Er Ying Zhong Zheng 新生儿硬肿症)

Sclerema neonatorum is characterized by inflammation of the underlying subcutaneous fat, manifested by skin patches that are cool and hardened. The hard and swollen sites are particularly prevalent in the lateral leg or thigh, cheek, and there is even difficulty in breathing.

This belongs to the category of Neonatal cold or five stiffen syndrome in TCM the *Zhu Bing Yuan Hou Lun. Tai Han* (.General Treatise on the Causes and Symptoms of Diseases) 610 says: "When the woman is pregnant, she has excessive cold, it invades the uterus, resulting in neonatal cold." The incidence rate is higher in the winter. In modern view, the main cause of this illness is cold, though other factors include prematurity, low birth weight, asphyxia, and severe infection. Its pathogenesis may be related to temperature regulation of the newborn's central nervous system that is imperfectly developed and the characteristics of neonatal subcutaneous fat composition. The disease mainly occurs in the winter and cold seasons. The incidence occurs primarily in premature infants. The mild condition has a good prognosis, but severe cases have a high mortality rate.

Etiology and Pathology

The causes of the illness are congenital yang vacuity, incorrect care that results in increased yang vacuity manifesting as low body temperature, cold extremities, and stiffness of the body. The main pathogenesis is internal cold due to yang vacuity, and stasis of qi and blood.

Patterns

Yang Vacuity

This is caused by congenital vacuity, original yang vacuity with invasion of external cold, failure of warming the skin and muscles resulting in the slerema.

Blood stagnation due to cold invasion

When the body is invaded by cold it leads to retardation of Qi and blood circulation, so that it fails to warm the skin and muscles resulting in sclerema.

Diagnosis

- The newborn has a cold body with stiffening of the skin and muscles, no appetite, no crying, slow reaction.
- The body temperature is lower than 95° F(35°C).
- There is a history of difficulty or failure in keeping the body warm, premature birth or serious infection.

Diagnostic Notes

- The history of disease should focus on comprehensive inquiry, including whether or not the patient has a history of premature birth, dytsocia, twins, low birth weight, incorrect nursing and feeding, insufficient warming or inappropriate cold exposure and infectious diseases.
- Carefully palpate all areas, carefully palpate the legs, buttock, cheeks, upper limbs, abdomen and chest. The presence of hardness and temperature should be observed and noted related to the specific areas.
- The blood gas tension, blood sugar, electrolyte and renal function may be checked.
- Neonatal edema occurs commonly in physically weak children. The edema spreads over a wide range of the body, such as eye lids, scalp, limbs, there may be local hardness and swelling, cold skin that is dark and purple in color.

Neonatal period neonatal subcutaneous gangrene is a common characteristic of a severe infectious disease. Bacteria (mostly Staphylococcus aureus, pseudomonas aeruginosa) in the subcutaneous fat and connective tissue with lesions often occur in the lumbosacral region, back, and buttocks.

Keys to differentiation

The severity of sclerema neonatorum should be determined. Based on clinical manifestations, the disease can be divided into mild, moderate or severe. See the attached table.

Severity	Anus Temp.(F)	Axilla Temp.	Affected Area(%)	Function disorder of organs
Mild	≥95°	Negative	<20	no obvious
Moderate	<95°	0 or positive	25~50	refuse eating, no crying slow reaction, slow heart rate
Severe	<86°	negative	>50	shock, DIC, pneumorrhagia, renal failure

Note: The ranges are: head 20%, both upper limbs 18%, front chest and abdoman 14%, back and lumber and sacral 14%. Both lower limbs 26%. This is referring to the percentage of skin affected in each area.

Therapeutic Principle

Warm yang and expel cold, remove blood stasis open the channels, combined with an increasing hypothermia therapy for severe cases.

Pattern Differentiation

Yang Vacuity

Manifestation: very weak, entire body is cold to touch, inability to nurse or cry, rigidity of joints, pale and swollen skin and muscles, pale tongue, invisible index vein.

Treatment Principle Supplement qi and warm yang

Formula:

Shen Fu Tang (Radix Ginseng and Radix Aconiti Praeparata Decoction).
Ren Shen (Radix Ginseng) supplements original qi. Fu Zi (Radix Aconiti Praeparata) warms Yang. Huang Qi (Radix Astragali Membranaceus), Bai Zhu (Rhizoma Atractylodis) and Gui Zhi (Ramulus Cinnamomi Cassiae) may be added to supplement Qi, expel cold and open the channels.

Blood stasis due to cold invasion

Manifestation: Cold and hard skin and muscles. It starts in the legs and gradually develops to the buttocks and cheeks, pale and purple tongue, deep and stagnated index vein.

Treatment method: expel cold and open the channels

Formula: Dang Gui Si Ni Tang (Tang Kuei Decoction for Frigid Extremities).

Dang Gui (Radix Angelicae Sinensis Root) supplements blood and removes stasis, Bai Shao (Fried Radix Paeoniae Lactiflorae) supplements blood, Gui Zhi (Ramulus Cinnamomi Cassiae) and Xi Xin (Herba Cun Radicae Asari) are warming and open the channels. Gan Cao (Radix Glycyrrhizae Uralensis) and Da Zao (Frutus Jujubae) supplement the spleen qi. If the skin and muclses are very hard and purple, add Tao Ren (Semen Persicae), Hong Hua (Flos Carthami Tinctorii) and Dan Shen (Radix Salviae Miltiorrhizae) to quicken the blood and remove stasis.

Other therapy

External Therapy

- Fu Zi (Radix Aconiti Praeparata)60g, Gui Zhi (Ramulus Cinnamomi Cassiae)60g, Dan Shen (Radix Salviae Miltiorrhizae)30g, Gan Jiang (Rhizoma Zingiberis)30g.

Cook all of the herbs for about 30 minutes. The final amount of the prepared decoction is about 2000ml. The temperature of the decoction starts from 36°C then increases to 40°C. Let the infant soak in the decoction for 10~20minutes, 1~2times/day.

- Cong Bai (Bulbus Allii Fistulosi) 30g, Sheng Jiang (Rhizoma Zingiberis Recens) 30g and Dan Dou Chi (Semen Sojae Praeparatum)30g. Grind all of the three herbs, then fry it with add a little liquor until it is warm. Wrap it with cloth. Apply to the local areas topically, the temperature should be around 36~40°C

Prevention and Care

- Try to prevent a premature birth, avoid birth trauma, asphyxia and exposure to cold
- The temperature of the delivery room should be suitable and there should be good air circulation
- You can use a hot water bottle to warm local areas, but be careful not to overheat and damage the skin.

The Disorders of the umbilicus
(Qi Bu Ji Huan 脐部疾患)

Disorders of the umbilicus are caused by incorrect care of the umbilicus, underdevelopment of the umbilicus after birth, damp umbilicus, ulcers and hernia. The wet umbilicus is due to invasion of the umbilicus by water and dampness. The umbilical sore is due to invasion of umbilicus by damp-heat, manifested with reddish, swollen and painful umbilicus, or even with pus in the umbilicus. Umbilical hernia is due to the intestine moving out through umbilicus from the abdomen, manifested with crying and pain. You may visualize a bulge near the navel or it may appear as if the umbilicus is swollen.

The disorders of umbilicus were noted during the Sui dynasty (*Zhu Bing Yuan Hou Lun. Qi Chuan* (General Treatise on the Causes and Symptoms of Diseases) 610 says: "Umbilical sore is due to an infant's umbilicus not being dried properly after birth, in addition, the invasion of wind in the umbilicus, which is difficult to be cured. If it is not cured in time, it may result in epilepsy". This means the cause, symptoms and treatment of the disorders were discussed in ancient medical books.

Etiology and Pathology

The main causes of this disorder are incorrect care of the umbilicus and thin, loose muscles of the abdominal wall due to congenital underdevelopment.

Diagnosis

- Umbilical moisture: moist umbilicus, exudation from the umbilicus
- Umbilical Sore: There is a history of improper care of the umbilical cord or there was an injury to the umbilical cord. It manifests with umbilical redness, swelling. oozing, pus, erosion and fever.
- Umbilical hernia: shiny and round swelling of the umbilicus. this becomes more obvious when the infant cries.

Diagnostic Notes

The umbilicus should be carefully observed. Note redness, swelling, secretions, and protrusion of the umbilicus.

Note all accompanying signs and symptoms.

Differential Diagnosis

Both umbilical intestinal fistula and umbilical urethral fistula are located at the umbilicus. There may be secretions of fluids. It is necessary, if available to perform X-rays to help confirm the diagnosis.

Pattern Differentiation

Differentiate between mild and severe symptoms. If the condition is mild, manifestations will be local to the umbilical cord without systemic involvement. If the condition is severe there may be fever, anxiety, convulsions, coma, umbilical redness and ulcerations of the umbilicus. These will all be in addition to the local symptoms at the umbilicus.

Umbilical dampness

Manifestations: sticky fluid from the umbilicus, as result, the umbilical region is wet, and slightly swollen.

Treatment Principle Dry dampness and astringe fluids

Formula: Long Gu San (Os Draconis Powder).

Long Gu (Os Draconis) and Ku Fan(Alumen Praeparatum) dry damp and generate tissue. These are used externally in the affected area. If the umbilicus is red and swollen, Jin Huang San (Golden Yellow Powder) can be used externally in the local area to clear heat and dry dampness.

Umbilical Sore

Manifestations: Redness, swelling, erosion, and pus oozing from the umbilicus. There may be high fever, crying and agitation if the case is severe.

Treatment Principle Clear heat and resolve toxin.

Formula: Wu Wei Xiao Du Yin (Five Ingredient Decoction to Eliminate Toxin)

Jin Yin Hua (Honeysuckle Flower),Pu Gong Ying (Herbal Taraxaci Mongolici Cum Radice), Zi Hua Di Ding (Herba Cum Radice Violae Yedoensitis),Ye Ju Hua (Flos Chrysanthmi Indici), Zi Bei

Tian Kui (Herba Begoniae Fimbristipulatae) clear heat and resolve toxin. If the patient has constipation, add Da Huang (Radix et Rhizoma Rhei) to drain heat.

Umbilical hernias

Manifestations: shiny, round swelling of the umbilicus, which can be pressed into the abdomen and protrudes when the infant cries or coughs.

Treatment method: It can close automatically in 3 months if the entire umbilical hernia is small. Laying supine may promote natural healing. Hernias measuring 2-5cm in diameter can be observed up to 2 years old and then surgical repair should be considered.

Other therapy

Patent herb Xiao Er Hua Du San (Detoxification Powder) 0.2g/time, 2times/day. It has the function of clearing heat and detoxification. It is used for umbilical hernias.

Acupuncture St25, Ren6, Ren3, Tituo, St36, Ren9, Du20. Perform once a day for two weeks as one course of treatment. This is used for umbilical hernias.

Topical treatment

Jin Huang San (Golden Yellow Powder) 1~2g, mixed with water as paste. Put it on the umbilicus, once a day. This is used for umbilical sore.

Bing Peng San (Borneol and Borac Powder) 1g topically used on umbilicus for umbilical dampness and sore.

Hai Piao Xiao (Cuttlefish Bone) 3g, grind and mix with sesame oil. Put it on the affected area for umbilical sores.

Prevention and Care

- The neonatal umbilicus is cut under strictly sterile conditions.
- Maintain cleanliness of the neonatal umbilicus, clean and dry to prevent infection.
- Underwear and diaper contact of the newborn should be soft to avoid scratching the skin.
- Frequently changes the diapers to avoid of umbilicus having frequent contact with urine
- Frequently observe the umbilicus. If there is exudate, treat immediately. If there is an umbilical hernia, the crying and coughing should be controlled.

If umbilical sores are serious and are accompanied by other complications, all of them should be treated promptly.

Diseases of the
Respiratory System

The diseases and syndromes of the respiratory system are located primarily in the lungs, however mechanisms may co-exist or originate from other body systems. The lung is located in the chest. Internally the lung meridian travels upwards connecting with the airway and throat and opens into the nose. The lung is called the Huagai, or florid canopy. The lung is the anatomically most superior of all the zang fu organs. They protect the other organs from invasion of exogenous pathogenic factors. The structure of the lung is like an empty beehive and acts like a bellows in the body. The physiological function of the lung is to control qi, perform respiration, coordinating visceral activities and regulation of the body's metabolism. The lung's primary physiological function is the dispersion and downbearing of qi. The syndromes of respiration are likely caused by failure in this function. To disperse and downbear the lung qi is the most common therapy in TCM pediatrics. The lung's relationship to other organs should also be carefully considered when devising a treatment plan. For example, there is the mother-son relationship between the spleen and lung, respectively. If the spleen fails to transport and transform it generates phlegm that is stored in the lungs. We can treat this by supplementing the mother spleen in order to improve the lung function. The lung controls the qi, respiration, and metabolism. The kidney controls water metabolism and regulates qi. Therefore disorders of water and breath are likely related to lung and kidney function. The lung coordinates visceral activities. The heart controls blood and blood circulation, therefore the circulation of qi and blood rely on the normal function of the lung and heart. This relationship must be considered when the lung is dysfunctional. The disorders of the lung are quite common and often critical and complicated. The characteristics of pulmonary diseases are likely to: include heat mechanisms, to be complicated, to change rapidly and include qi and yin vacuity.

The general treatment of this system is to disperse lung qi and downbear qi. In addition, the following methods should be used appropriately.

- Clear heat from the lung, nourish lung yin and moisten the lung.
- Treat the related organs and concurrent mechanisms.
- Actively prevent complications and changeability of pulmonary diseases.

Common Cold (Gan Mao 感冒)

The common cold is a pulmonary illness that is caused by the invasion of exterior pathogens due to inadequate clothing, sudden change of weather, constitutional weakness, and insufficiency of defensive qi. It presents with fever, chills, stuffy nose, sneezing, runny nose, and cough. It is also named as Shang Feng (Wind Damage) or Shang Feng Gan Mao (Comon cold due to Wind damage) is named as such because wind is the primary vehicle which ushers these pathogenic factors into the body. Most of the symptoms of common cold are likely located in the head and lung.

Gan Mao includes the common cold and influenza. The common cold is caused by the invasion of the six evils in the four seasons. Influenza is caused by infection and can become epidemic. The symptoms of the flu are much more severe. All ages of patients may suffer from this disease, but the incidence is much higher among infants. It often occurs in the fall and spring, especially when there is a sudden climate change.

Etiology and Pathology

These diseases occur with inappropriate clothing and pathogenic evils invade the exterior from the skin and mouth. They enter into the lung and disrupt Wei qi. It manifests with aversion to cold or heat, fever and chills, nasal congestion, runny nose, sneezing, headache, general discomfort and cough. Because physiological and pathological features of children are different from that of adults, the following are the most common characteristics of the common cold in children.

- *Heat syndromes.* Because the constitution of children is pure Yang, their diseases are easy to transform quickly into ones of heat and fire.
- *Phlegm.* The lung in children is especially delicate. When pathogens invade the body, the dispersing and downbearing function of the lung is inhibited. The fluid accumulates in the lung and transforms into phlegm resulting in a patient whose cough will be severe. There will commonly be shortness of breath as well.
- *Food Stagnation.* In children, the spleen is weak. The stomach is small and tender and is not capable of dealing with large amounts of food. If the exterior evils invade the lung, this will disrupt the transformation and transportation function of the spleen and stomach. This will lead to food stagnation presenting as abdominal fullness, low appetite, vomiting and diarrhea.
- *Convulsions.* The liver and the heart tend to surplus. When children suffer from the invasion of exterior evils, these patterns are likely to transform into fire, stirring up wind causing convulsions. This manifests as irritability, anxiety, crying, grinding teeth at night, easily frightened and finally convulsions.

Diagnosis

Diagnostic Guidelines

The main manifestations are aversion to cold and heat, chills and fever, nasal stuffiness, runny nose, sneezing, cough, reddish throat, floating pulse and index vein. If all of the above are severe then we should consider influenza. If there is a history of inappropriate clothing or sudden climate change, we should consider the common cold.

Additional points of diagnosis

- *Measles*: In addition to the symptoms of the common cold we may also see Koplik's spots and rashes.
- *Chickenpox*: A rash occurs about 10 to 21 days after initial exposure. The child develops small, itchy, fluid-filled blisters and red spots all over the body.
- *Exanthema Subitum*: This generally occurs in children under two years of age. The symptoms are usually limited to a transient rash that occurs following a fever that lasts about three days. After a few days the fever subsides, and just as the child appears to be recovering, a red rash appears.
- *Infantile pneumonia*: The patient may have chills and fever, runny nose, sore throat, cough, which are all symptoms similar to the common cold. However, this disease includes a higher fever, labored breathing, wheezing, flaring nostrils and chest retractions. Chest retractions are described as a sucking in of the skin around the bones upon inhalation.

Diagnostic Notes

- The history of the disease should be inquired and clearly understood.
- The accompanying symptoms should be carefully considered.
- The throat and any rashes should be inspected carefully. Submaxillary lymph nodes should be palpated. The heart and lungs should be auscultated.

Pattern Differentiation

Guidelines of differentiation

Differentiating between cold and heat

In order for us to conclude that the pattern differentiation is due to wind-cold the patient must present with chills greater than fever, thick nasal discharge, and a red and swollen throat. If there is fever with turbid phlegm, red and swollen throat, a red tongue, a tongue coating that is thin, yellow and dry, then a wind-heat pattern is present. If there is aversion to cold and a runny nose, it is mostly due to a complex of cold and heat or cold transforming into heat. If the onset occurs during the summer with high fever, none or slight sweating, thirst, and irritability it is due to summer-heat. If there is severe aversion to chills, runny nose, clear phlegm, pink tongue with a thin, white coating, then invasion of cold is present.

Differentiating between the common cold and influenza

In order to effectively differentiate between a common cold and the flu, the severity of the symptoms are carefully considered, and whether or not it is epidemic. If there are fever and chills, a mild cough, then it is most likely a common cold. If these symptoms are more severe and there is widespread infection you should consider influenza.

Differentiation of complex syndromes

If the case is complicated with a heavy cough and phlegm there is a concurrent phlegm syndrome. If there is loss of appetite, diarrhea or constipation, and vomiting then food stagnation is present. If there is irritability, crying, grinding teeth at night, fearfulness, palpitations or even convulsions it indicates convulsion.

Therapeutic Principles

Expelling the pathogen and releasing the exterior is the most common therapy. Releasing the exterior with acrid and warm herbs is appropriate for wind-cold patterns, while wind-heat patters respond when acrid and cool herbs are used properly. Using medicinals that release the exterior and clear summer-heat are appropriate in the treatment of summer-heat. If there is phlegm add medicinals that disperse the lung and resolve phlegm. If there is food stagnation, include herbs to assist the digestion. If there are convulsions, use medicinals to calm the spirit and extinguish liver wind.

Patterns and Treatment

Wind-cold

Manifestations

chills greater than fever, aversion to cold, thick and clear phlegm, runny nose, sneezing, headache, red and swollen throat

Treatment principle Release exterior, expel cold with warm, acrid herbs

Formula

Cong Chi Tang is used for a mild wind-cold invasion. Jing Fang Bai Du San (Schizonepeta and Ledebouriella Antiphlogistic Powder) is used for more severe cases. Jing Fang Bai Du San (Schizonepeta and Ledebouriella Antiphlogistic Powder) is used for severe wind cold. Jing Jie (Herbs Seu Flos Schizonepetae Tenuifoliae), Fang Feng (Redix Ledebouriella Divaricatae), Sheng Jiang (Rhizoma Zinggiberis Officinalis Recens), Chai Hu (Radix Bupleuri) and Bo He (Herba Menthae haplocalycis) expel exterior syndrome and relieve fever. Chuan Xiong (Radix Ligustici Chuanxiong) removes blood stasis, expels wind and stops pain. Jie Geng (Radix Platycodi Grandifori), Zhi Ke(Bitter Orange Peel), Fu Ling(Sclerotium Poria Cocos) and Gan Cao (Radix Glycyrrhizae Uralensis) for disperse and regulate lung Qi, and resolve phlegm. Du Huo (Radix Angelicae Pubescentis) and Qiang Huo (Rhizoma et Radix Notopterygii) expel wind cold. Jin Yin Hua (Flos Lonicerae Japonicae) and Lian

Qiao (Fructus Forsythiae Suspensae), are used if the fever is worse due to exterior wind cold turning to heat.

Jing Jie (Herbs Seu Flos Schizonepetae Tenuifoliae), Fang Feng (Redix Ledebouriella Divaricatae), Sheng Jiang (Rhizoma Zinggiberis Officinalis Recens), Chai Hu (Radix Bupleuri) and Bo He (Herba Menthae Haplocalycis) expel cold, release the exterior and relieve fever. Chuan Xiong (Radix Ligustici Chuanxiong) quickens blood stasis, expels wind and relieves pain. Jie Geng (Radix Platycodi Grandifori), Zhi Ke(Bitter Orange Peel), Fu Ling (Sclerotium Poria Cocos) and Gan Cao(Radix Glycyrrhizae Uralensis) disperse and downbear lung qi and resolve phlegm. Du Huo (Radix Angelicae Pubescentis) and Qiang Huo (Rhizoma et Radix Notopterygii) expel wind-cold. If the fever increases due to cold transforming into heat. add Jin Yin Hua (Flos Lonicerae Japonicae) and Lian Qiao (Fructus Forsythiae Suspensae),

Wind-heat

Manifestations

aversion to heat slight chills, headache, malaise, sneezing, cough, thick and yellow phlegm, reddish and swollen throat, red tongue with a thin, yellow coat, floating and rapid pulse or floating purple index vein.

Treatment Principle Clear heat, expel wind and release exterior with cool and acrid herbs

Formula

Yin Qiao San (Honeysuckle and Forsythia Powder)
Jin Yin Hua (Honeysuckle Flower) and Lian Qiao (Forsythia Fruit) expel wind-heat with their pungent flavor and cool nature while their aromatic properties clear turbidness and toxin. Bo He (Herba Menthae Haplocalycis) and Niu Bang Zi (Arctium Fruit) and Jie Geng (Platycodon Root) expel wind-heat and soothe the throat. Dan Zhu Ye (Bamboo Leaf), Jing Jie (Schizonepeta), Dan Dou Chi (Prepared Soybean), Lu Gen (Rhizoma Phragmitis

Communis)) and Gan Cao(Licorice) clear wind-heat. If the fever is severe, add Shi Gao (Gypsum), Yu Xing Cao (Houttuynia Cordata), Huang Qin (Radix Scutellariae Baicalensis) and Zhi Zi (Fructus Gardeniae). If the patient has reddish and sore throat, Niu Bang Zi (Fructus Arctii Lappae) and She Gan (Belamcanda Chinesis) can be added. If there is epistaxis, Bai Mao Gen (Rhizoma Imperatae Cylidricae) and Xian He Cao (Herba Agrimoniae Pilosae) are added.

Summer-heat

Manifestations

aversion to heat without fever, chest distention, abdominal distention, poor appetite, vomiting, diarrhea

Treatment Principle Release exterior, clear heat, drain dampness

Formula

Xin Jia Xiang Ru Yin (Newly Augmented Elsholtzia Decoction)
Xiang Ru (Herba Elsholtziae Seu Moslae) expels summer-heat and dampness. Jin Yin Hua (Honeysuckle flower) and Lian Qiao (Forsythia Fruit) and Bai Bian Dou (Semen Dolichos Lablab) clear heat and drain dampness. Hou Po (Cortex Magnoliae Officinalis) drains dampness and relieves abdominal fullness. If the patient also has Yangming heat, then add Bai Hu Tang (White Tiger Decoction). If there is crying and anxiety caused by heat in the heart, add Dan Zhu Ye (Herba Loptatheri Gracilis) and Lian Xin (Nelumbinis nuciferae). If there is severe abdominal fullness and poor appetite add Cang zhu (Rhizoma Atractylodis) and Yi Yi Ren (Coix Lachryma-jobi) to drain dampness and harmonize the middle.

Complications

Food Stagnation

In addition to the symptoms of common cold there may be poor appetite, vomiting of sour food, coating. The treatment principle includes promoting digestion and relieving stagnation. Shan Zha (Frutus Crataegi), Mai Ya (Fructus Hordei Vulgaris Germinantus), Shen Qu (Massa fermentata), Gu Ya (Fructus Oryzae Sativae Germinantus) and Ji Nei Jin(Endithelium Corneum) can be added for food stagnation. If the patient has constipation, yellow and scanty urine, rough and turbid tongue coating add Da Huang (Radix et Rhizoma Rhei), Zhi Shi (Fructus Immaturus Citri Aurantii) and Bing Lang (Semen Arecae Catechu) to purge the food stagnation.

Convulsions

In addition to the above symptoms of common cold there may be convulsions, fright, crying, restlessness, teeth grinding, red tongue, wiry pulse or purple index vein. The treatment principle is to clear heat, release the exterior, calm the spirit and extinguish wind. Chan Tui (Periostracum Cicadae) and Gou Teng (Ramulus cum uncis uncariae) can be added.

Other treatment

Patents

- Xiao Chai Hu Ke Li (Minor Buplureum Granule). Take this orally, 1 package TID. It is used for common cold with alternating chills and fever.
- Xia Er Hui Chuan Dan (Spring Back Pill for Children). Taken orally, use 1 package TID. This is used for common cold with convulsions.
- Chai Hu Zhu She Yi (Buplureum Injection). Drip into the nose, 2~3 drops per nostril every 1~2 hours. It is used for the common cold with high fever.

Prevention and care

- Take part in outdoor activities getting adequate sun exposure. This can help to supplement the immune system.
- Pay attention to sudden and severe weather changes. Dress the child in layers that can be easily added or removed.

- Try to avoid public exposure when incidence of flu is high.
- Avoid eating too many foods that are too dry, cold, greasy and sweet. Give more water if the child has a cold and give foods that are easy to digest.

Susceptible Children

Some children are easy to catch colds. This is common in infants, and the incidence has increased in recent years. Many children aren't treated in time or are treated incorrectly. These factors can lead to pneumonia and asthma attacks. The most prevalent pathogenic factor with these children is spleen and lung qi vacuity and weak Wei qi. The treatment method in the remission stage is to supplement the qi and strengthen the exterior. To treat lung qi vacuity use Yu Ping Feng San (Jade Windscreen Powder) or Huang Qi Gui Zhi Wu Wu Tang (Astragalus and Cinnamon Twig Five Substance Decoction). If there is spleen qi vacuity use Shen Ling Bai Zhu San (Ginseng, Poria, Atractylodes and Macrocephala Powder). When illness is present everyone should increase hand-washing, especially before eating and after going outside. Make sure to dress appropriately for the weather and be prepared for sudden weather changes. Eat a balanced diet.

Tonsillitis (Ru E 乳蛾)

Tonsillitis is a pulmonary disorder that is characterized by reddish, swollen tonsils that may or may not have white patches, and a sore throat. Tonsillitis is called Ru E in China, Ru E translates as silk moth. This refers to the lacy, white patches that may form on the tonsils. If there is unilateral swelling in the throat it is called Dan Ru E (single silk moth). If the throat is swollen bilaterally it is called Shuang Ru E (double silk moth). If pus is present on the tonsils then it is called Lan Ru E (rotten silk moth).

Chong Lou Yu Yue says "it is caused by an accumulation of heat in the lung with attack of exogenous pathogenic factors. Any or all of these can present as tonsils swollen like a "silk moth". This can occur in any season, symptoms can be severe or mild. Severity can be due to age or strength of defensive qi. The prognosis is positive after treatment, but there can be complications such as edema, palpitations, Bi syndrome and Otitis Media due to incorrect or untimely treatment.

Etiology and Pathology

The throat is the gateway of the lung and stomach. There are two primary mechanisms causing tonsillitis. Exogenous evils may invade the lung or chronic stomach heat may disturb the stomach and lung. Heat and toxins rise upward into the throat and mouth causing this disease.

Diagnosis

Diagnostic Guidelines

The main manifestations include swollen and red tonsils, itching throat, pus on the tonsils. In mild cases there may not be accompanying symptoms, when severe there will be fever, chills headache, body aches and cough.

Differential diagnosis

- Common cold: fever and chills, nasal congestion, runny nose, sneezing, cough, swollen and red throat
- Thrush: this manifests with white patches inside the oral cavity and on the tongue. There is fever and swollen, red throat.

Diagnostic Notes

- The symptoms of tonsillitis include fever, cough, difficulty breathing and vomiting must be addressed initially.
- The color, size, shape or the tonsils should be observed as well as whether pus is present.

- The conditions of the joints, urine and heart should be considered in older children, because it may cause rheumatic arthritis, nephritis and myocarditis.
- If the tonsils are red, swollen, purulent with systemic accompanying symptoms then blood work should be ordered, which indicates there is a severe infection. Refer this case to their family physician.

Pattern Differentiation

Guidelines of Differentiation

First, the severity of the condition needs to be assessed. If the disease occurs slowly, mild swelling of the tonsils with no pus, and there is little or no fever then this is mild tonsillitis. On the other hand if onset is sudden with severely swollen tonsils containing pus, high fever and other systemic symptoms this is severe tonsillitis.

Differentiate between vacuity and repletion. If the disease is of a relatively short duration with severely red and swollen tonsils, pus, accompanying systemic symptoms, a red tongue with a yellow coat this is a repletion pattern. If the syndrome occurred gradually and has been present for a longer time and all symptoms are relatively mild then this is a vacuity pattern, or a combination of vacuity and repletion.

Therapeutic Principles

The basic principle is to clear heat and relieve toxicity, reduce swelling and benefit the throat. If the mechanism is wind-heat, medicinals to clear heat and expel wind should be added. If there is excessive heat and toxin, medicinals to clear heat toxin and purge fire are used. If there is yin vacuity of the lung and stomach, add medicinals to nourish lung and stomach yin.

Patterns and Treatment

Wind-heat Invasion

Manifestations

swollen and red tonsils, itchy throat, fever, mild chills, runny nose, headache, body aches, red tongue with thin and yellow coating, floating and rapid pulse, purple index vein.

Treatment Principle Expel wind, clear heat, reduce swelling, benefit throat

Formula

Yin Qiao Ma Bo San (honeysuckle, forsythia and puffball powder)
    Jin Yin Hua (Flos Lnicerae Japonicae) and Lian Qiao (Fructus Forsythiae Suspensae) clear heat and expel wind. She Gan Belamcanda Chinesis), Niu Bang Zi(Fructus Arctii) and Ma Bo (Lasiosphaera Fenslii) benefit the throat and reduce swelling. If tonsils are severely swollen add Ban Lan Gen (Radix Isatidis Seu Baphicacanthi) to resolve toxin and benefit the throat. If fever is high, Shi Gao (Gypsum), Lu Gen (Rhizoma Phargmitis, Huang Qin (Radix Scutellariae Baicalensis) and Zhi Zi (Fructus Gardeniae) can be added to clear heat and resolve toxin. If the patient has hoarseness add, Pi Pa Ye (Eriobotryae Japobicae) and. Chan Tui (Periostracum Cicadae) to disperse the lung Qi and benefit the throat.

Toxic-heat invasion

Manifestations: severely swollen and red tonsils with pus, high fever, thirst, bad breath, red tongue with thick and yellow coating, rapid pulse, purple index vein.

Treatment Principle

clear heat, resolve toxin, reduce swelling, benefit the throat.

Formula

Niu Bang Gan Jie Tang (Arctium fruit, Glycyrrhizae Uralensis and Radix Platycodi Grandifori Decoction)

Niu Bang Zi (Fructus Arctii Lappae), Shan Dou Gen (Ophora Subprotrata), She Gan(Belamcanda Chinesis), Jie Gen(Radix Platycodi Grandiflori), Xuan Shen (Radix Scrophulariae Ningpoensis) resolove toxin and benefit the throat. Huang Lian (Rhizoma Coptidis), Huang Qin (Radix Scutellariae Baicalensis), Zhi Zi (Fructus Gardeniae Jasminoidis), Gan Cao (Radix Glycyrrhizae Uralensis) to clear heat and resolve toxin. If patient has high fever add Shi Gao (Gypsum) and Zhi Mu (Rhizome Anemarrhenae). If there is severe pus on the tonsils add, Jin Yin Hua (Flos Lonicerae Japonicae), Yu Xing Cao (Houttuynia Cordata) and Pu Gong Ying (Herba Taraxaci Mongolici Cum) to resolve toxin and expel pus. If the tonsils and tongue are deep red add, Mu Dan Pi (Cortex Moutan Radicis), Sheng Di Huang (Radix Rehmanniae Glutinosae) and Chi Shao (Radix Paeoniae Rubra) to clear heat and cool the blood. If patient has restlessness, irritability, or even convulsion of limbs add, Gou Teng (Ramulus Cum Uncis Uncariae) Chan Tui (Periostracum Cicadae), Di Long (Lumbricus) to expel wind and calm the liver.

Yin vacuity of the lung and stomach

Manifestations

chronic red and swollen tonsils with dry and itching throat, dry cough with little phlegm, constipation and scanty urination, red tongue with scanty coating, thin and rapid pulse or purple index vein

Treatment Principle Generate Yin and nourish the lung, benefit throat and resolve swelling

Formula

Yang Yin Qing Fei Tang (Nourish the yin and clear the lung decoction). Xuan Shen (Radix scrophulariae Ningpoensis), Mai

Men Dong (ophiopogon root), and Sheng Di Huang (uncooked Radix Rehmanniae) nourish Yin and benefit the throat. Mu Dan Pi (Cortex Mountan Radicis), Bai Shao (Radix Paeoniae Lactiflorae) cool the blood. Bei Mu (Bulbus Fritillariae), Bo He (Herba Menthae Haplocalycis), and Gan Cao (Licorice Root) clear heat and benefit the throat. If the patient has a swollen throat add, Xia Ku Cao (Spica Prunella Vulgaris), Niu Bang Zi (Fructus Arctii) and Hai Zao (Herba Sargassii) to benefit the throat and resolve phlegm. If there is hoarseness add, He Zi (Fructus Terminaliae Chebulae) and Er Cha (Pasta Acaciae Seu Uncaruae) to benefit the throat.

Other Treatment

Ready-made formulas

- Xi Gua Shuang Run Hou Pian (Watermelon Frost Lozenges) 1pill/time, frequently keeping in the mouth. It is used for wind- heat or Yin vacuity of lung and stomach.
- Bing Peng San (Borneol and Borax Powder) Blown into the throat. It is used for excessive heat and toxin of school children.

Prevention and care

- Pay attention to oral hygiene, active prevention of dental caries
- Prevent and treat colds.
- Avoid eating spicy or dry foods
- Try to cure the disease in time and prevent protracted illness or other concurrent disease

Cough (Ke Sou 咳嗽)

Cough is one of the symptoms of pulmonary disorders. Ke means it has only one voice, without phlegm; Sou means it only has phlegm, but no voice. It is considered Ke Sou if there is both voice and phlegm. It is said "disorders of the five zang and six fu organs may result in cough. A cough is not strictly a disorder of the lungs, but is related to the lungs. *You You Ji Cheng* (Collection of Pediatrics) 1750 states "the Sou mainly results from phlegm and the treatment should focus on the spleen. The Ke that is without phlegm arises primarily from the lungs." Cough often occurs in winter and spring. The prognosis for most coughs is good, but some may be a symptom of deeper disease.

Etiology and Pathology

Children's lungs are particularly tender, their skin is soft and defensive qi is weak. This makes children more prone to suffering from exterior pathogenic factors. Therefore, children's cough results more often from exterior syndromes than interior. The location of the cough is in the lung, disrupting the dispersing and descending of lung qi.

Exterior pathogens attacking the lung

When wind invades the lungs through the nose and skin, the lung qi fails to disperse and descend resulting in cough. The wind is the carrier of all evils. It is the first to invade the body and other evils accompany wind. Wind is a yang pathogen. Children's constitutions are considered Pure Yang, therefore it is easy and common for wind invasion to transform into heat. Therefore, even a wind-cold invasion will quickly transform to heat, resulting in phlegm-heat accumulating in the lungs.

Phlegm generated from the interior

A child's spleen is generally regarded as weak. If kids are nursed and fed inappropriately this generates phlegm. Phlegm is generated by the spleen and is stored in the lungs. The phlegm will disrupt the dispersion and downbearing of the lung leading to cough.

Lung yin vacuity

Lung yin vacuity will occur as a result of lingering or chronic febrile disease. When lung yin fails to nourish the lung, lung qi will not adequately disperse and downbear leading to cough.

Diagnosis

Diagnostic Guidelines

- The main manifestations are cough with or without phlegm.
- The cough most commonly occurs with the common cold.

Diagnostic Notes

- The history should include the times when cough occurs, when it becomes worse, the frequency of the cough, the volume, color and odor of sputum as well as accompanying symptoms.
- The throat and nose should be observed
- The sound of the cough and the breath should be auscultated
- If there is fever or the cough is of a longer duration, then blood work, chest X-ray and sputum culture are indicated.

Pattern Differentiation

Guidelines of Differentiation

- Differentiate between internal and external patterns. External patterns typically include cough that has an acute onset, short history, fever, chills, and runny nose. Internal patterns typically include a cough that is chronic, enduring and accompanying symptoms that include other organ systems.
- Differentiate between cold, heat, vacuity and repletion. Exterior coughs are repletion patterns, interior coughs are vacuity patterns. Cough with clear sputum, a pale tongue with a white coat are due to cold patterns. While a cough that includes yellow sputum, a red tongue with a yellow coat or a peeled coat is caused by a heat pattern.

Therapeutic Principle

The basic treatment principle is to disperse and descend lung qi. Releasing the exterior is appropriate for cough due to attack of external evils. In the case of interior patterns of cough the treatment principle is to dry damp, clear heat and nourish lung yin.

Patterns and Treatment

Exterior Cough

Wind-cold

Manifestations

Frequent cough with clear phlegm, itching throat, runny nose with clear discharge, chills without sweating, headache, body ache, white tongue coating, tight and floating pulse.

Treatment Principle Expel wind-cold, eliminate phlegm, disperse lung and descend qi, stop cough

Formula

Xing Su San (Apricot Kernel and Perilla Leaf Powder)
    Zi Su Ye (Folium Perillae Frutescentis) and Qian Hu (Radix Peucedani) disperse lung Qi and releases exterior. Jie Geng (Radix Platycodi Grandiflori) and Xing Ren (Semen Pruni Armeniacae) descend lung Qi. Ban Xia (Rhizoma Pinelliae Terntae), Fu Ling (Sclerotium Poria Cocos), Zhi Ke (Fructus Immaturus Citri Aurantii) and Chen Pi (Pericarpium Citri Reticulatae) eliminate phlegm, dry dampness and descend lung Qi. Gan Cao (Radix Glycyrrhizae Uralensis), Sheng Jiang (Rhizoma Zingiberis Recens) and Da Zao (Fructus Zizyphy Jujubae) harmonize Ying and Wei. If the patient has a sore throat, hoarseness, and thirst due to exterior cold and interior heat, Yu Xing Cao (Houttuynia Cordata), Pi Pa Ye (Eriobotryae Japobicae) and Huang Qin (Radix Scutellariae Baicalensis) can be added to clear heat.

Wind-heat

Manifestations

Cough with yellow, sticky sputum that is difficult to expectorate, sore throat, yellow nasal discharge, fever, thirst, red tongue with thin and yellow coating, floating and rapid pulse or floating and purple index vein.

Treatment Principle Expel wind and clear heat, disperse lung and descend qi, stop cough

Formula

Sang Ju Yin (Mulberry Leaf and Chrysanthemum Decoction)

Sang Ye (Mulberry Leaf), Ju Hua (Chrysanthemum Flower), Bo He (Herba Menthae Haplocalycis) and Lian Qiao (Forsythia Fruit) expel evil and clear lung heat to relieve cough. Xing Ren (Bitter Apricot Kernel), Jie Geng (Platycodon Root) eliminate phlegm and relieve cough. Lu Gen (Reed Rhizome), Gan Cao(Licorice) clear heat.

Ma Xing Shi Gan Tang (Ephedra, Apricot, Licorice and Gypsum Decoction) can be added into this formula for the patient who has severe cough due to phlegm-heat in the lungs. If the fever is high, Shi Gao (Gypsum), Yu Xing Cao (Houttuynia Cordata), Huang Qin (Radix Scutellariae Baicalensis) and Zhi Zi (Fructus Gardeniae) can be added to clear heat and toxin. If there is cough with a lot of phlegm, Qian Hu (Radix Peucedani), Gua Lou (Peel Fructus Trichosanthis), Tian Zhu Huang (Bambusa Textilis) are added to clear heat and eliminate phlegm. If the patient has a severely red and sore throat, Niu Bang Zi (Fructus Arctii Lappae), She Gan (Belamcanda Chinesis) can be added to clear heat toxin and soothe the throat If the patient also has anxiety and night crying, Chan Tui (Periostracum Cicadae) and Gou Teng (Ramulus Cum Uncis Uncariae) can be added to extinguish wind and calm night terrors.

Damp-heat

Manifestations

Coughing with a lot of phlegm, sore throat, runny nose with sticky discharge, poor appetite, abdominal fullness, nausea, vomiting, red tongue with yellow and greasy coating, a soft and floating pulse

Treatment Principle

clear heat and eliminate dampness, disperse lung and descend qi, stop cough

Formula

Shang Jiao Xuan Bi Tang (Dispersing Bi of Upper Jiao Decoction) Pi Pa Ye (Eriobotryae Japobicae), She Gan (Belamcanda Chinesis) and Dan Dou Chi (Semen Sojae Praeparatum) clear heat and disperse lung Qi, Yu Jin (Tuber Curcumae) regulate Qi and resolve stagnation, Tong Cao (Tetrapanax Papyriferus) clears damp heat. If chest distention and poor appetite are severe add Wei Jing Tang (Reed Decoction) to eliminate dampness and disperse lung Qi. If the cough is severe add Ma Xing Shi Gan Tang (Ephedra, Apricot, Licorice and Gypsum Decoction) to disperse lung qi and eliminate phlegm.

Interior cough

Phlegm-heat

Manifestations

Cough with a lot of yellow, sticky sputum that is difficult to expectorate, fever, irritability, yellow urine, constipation, red tongue with yellow coating, slippery and rapid pulse, or purple index vein

Treatment Principle Clear heat and purge lung, disperse lung and descend qi, stop cough

Formula

Qing Qi Hua Tan Tang (Clear Qi and Transform Phlegm Decoction)
Zhi Zi (Fructus Gardeniae Jasminoidis), Huang Qin (Radix Scutellariae Baicalensis), Zhi Mu (Rhizome Anemarrhenae) clear heat and purge the lung, Sang Bai Pi (Cortex Mori Albae Radicis) and Gua Lou (Fructus Trichosanthis), Zhe Bei Mu (Fritillaria Thunbergii), Chen Pi (Pericarpium Citri Reticulatae) disperse the lung qi and expel phlegm, Fu Ling (Sclerotium Poria Cocos) supplements the spleen and eliminates phlegm, Mai Men Dong (Ophiopogon Root), Jie Geng (Radix Platycodi Grandifori) and Gan Cao (Licorice Root) moisten the lungs and eliminate phlegm. Sha Shen (Radix Adenophorae Strictae) and Di Gu Pi (Cortex Lycii Radicis) are recommended for nourishing Yin and clearing heat if the tongue is red with a glossy coating. Mu Dan Pi (Cortex Moutan Radicis), Bai Mao Gen (Rhizoma Imperatae Cylidricae) cool the blood and stop bleeding.

Phlegm-damp

Manifestations

Cough with copious, thin and clear phlegm, chest fullness, poor appetite, fatigue heavy and tired, pale tongue with white and slippery coating, slippery pulse

Treatment Principle Dry dampness and eliminate phlegm, disperse lung Qi and downbear lung qi

Formula

Ma Xing Er Chen Tang (Ephedra, Apricot, two-Cured Decoction)
Ma Huang (Herba ephedra) and Xing Ren (Semen Pruni Armeniacae) disperse and downbear lung Qi, Er Chen Tang supplements Spleen and drains dampness. Su Zi (Perilla Frutescens), Che Qian Zi (Plantago Asiatica) are added to downbear lung Qi and expel phlegm if there is a lot of phlegm. Gan Jiang (Rhizoma Zingiberis), Xi Xin (Herba Cun Radicae Asari) are added if there

is severe cold and damp. If there is pale face and fatigue add Dang Shen (Radix Codonopsitis Pilosulae) and Bai Zhu (Rhizoma Atractylodis) to supplement spleen Qi. If there is food stagnation and poor appetite add Shan Zha (Frutus Crataegi), Mai Ya (Fructus Hordei Vulgaris Germinantus), Shen Qu (Massa Fermentata)

Yin vacuity

Manifestations

Slight cough, sticky phlegm, that is difficult to expectorate, dry throat, hoarseness, hot palms, night sweats, red lips and a tongue with glossy coating, thready and rapid pulse or purple index vein.

Treatment Principle

Nourish Yin and moisten lungs, eliminate phlegm and stop cough

Formula

Sha Shen Mai Dong Tang (Glehnia and Ophiopogonis Decoction)
    Sha Shen (Radix Adenophorae Strictae), Mai Men Dong (Tuber Ophiopogonis Japonici) and Yu Zhu (Rhizoma Polygonti Odorati) nourish Yin and clear the lungs, Sang Ye (Mulberry Leaf) clears heat, Bai Bian Dou (Dolichos Lablab) and Gan Cao (Radix Glycyrrhizae Uralensis) harmonize the middle Jiao. Tian Hua Fen (Radix Trichosanthes) generates yin. Qing Hao (Artemeisia Apiacea) claers heat. If there is a low-grade fever add Hu Huang Lian (Rhizoma Picrorrhizae). If there is poor appetite due to Stomach yin vacuity add Shan Zha (Frutus Crataegi) and Shi Wei (Folium Pyrrosia)

Ready-made Medicinals

- Zhu Li(Succus Bambusae): Taken orally for cough due to phlegm-heat. 3ml t.i.d. for children under three years old. 5ml t.i.d., for children older than 3 years old.
- Chuan Bei Pi Pa Tang Jiang (Bulus Fritillariae Cirrhosae and Loquat Syrup): Taken orally for cough due to Yin

vacuity. 3 ml t.i.d. for children under three years old. 5ml t.i.d., for children older than 3 years old. ·

Prevention and care

- Pay attention to weather changes and avoid over-exposure to cold weather.
- Avoid the food and habits that irritate the throat like acidic foods fatty foods, spicy foods, coarse foods, too much crying, shouting, cigarette smoke and dust.

Pneumonia (Fei Yan Chuan Sou 肺炎喘嗽)

Pneumonia is called Fei Yan Chuan Sou in Chinese. Fei means lung. Yan means inflammation in Chinese, however in TCM Yan refers to repletion heat. Chuan means wheezing and Sou means cough. Pneumonia manifests with fever, cough, shortness or breath and nostril flaring. The earliest mention of the term pneumonia was by Xie Yu Qiong, a physician in the Qing dynasty, in his book titled *Ma Ke Huo Ren Quan Shu* (Saving Life of Children Who Have Measles). He said the syndrome presented with movement of the shoulders during respiration, wheezing, nasal flaring. These are due to the replete heat in the lungs, a key symptom with pneumonia, that obstructs the dispersing and downbearing of the lung. Information about this syndrome can also be found in Fei Zhang (Lung distention) and Ma Pi Feng (Spleen wind of the Horse) previous to the Qing dynasty. Pneumonia occurs easily in infants and toddlers in all four seasons, but is most common in winter and spring. Usually the prognosis of pneumonia is good if it is treated early and properly. Though there can be complications such as exhaustion of heart yang, heat invading Jueyin and even death if treated incorrectly or if treatment is not initiated promptly. Infants or children, especially ones with a weak constitution, may have relapses or develop a chronic version of the disease.

Etiology and Pathology

There are three basic mechanisms that can lead to pneumonia. When the weather and temperature changes suddenly, the exterior pathogens invade the lungs through the skin, mouth and nose and can lead to pneumonia. The lung is invaded by pathogenic heat in the case of measles or pertussis. Or, while recovering from a recent illness, the patient is once again attacked by exogenous pathogens leading to pneumonia.

Suffering exterior pathogens, with evils blocking the lung

Exterior pathogens in body obstruct the lungs and lead to failure of the lung qi to descend, which leads to Fei Yan Chuan Sou. This can occur in a pattern of wind-heat or wind-cold. Wind-heat obstructing the lungs is more common in the clinic, because of children's constitutional features.

Excessive heat obstructing lung

The excessive heat obstructing the lung is caused by incorrect treatment at the early stage of disease or weak vital energy. This leads to phlegm-heat resulting from the heat burning fluids. Phlegm-heat then obstructs the lung resulting in typical manifestations of Fei Yan Chuan Sou, such as fever, cough, shortness of breath, nasal flaring and copious phlegm in the lung.

Exhaustion of heart Yang

Because the lungs govern qi and blood circulation of the entire body, if heat blocks the lung qi, blood flow will not be smooth. This creates blood stasis and can damage the heart. The lung fails to produce enough Zong qi (Pectoral/Ancestral qi), which is too weak to help the heart circulate the blood leading to heart qi vacuity, and even exhaustion of heart Yang. If both qi vacuity and blood stasis of the heart occur and are not treated in time heart yang will become exhausted. This manifests as a pale face, purple lips, palpitations, including the symptoms of pneumonia. Infants and those with a weak constitution or children whose weight is lower than normal suffer easily from exhaustion of heart Yang at an early stage.

Heat invading Jueyin

If heat is replete, heat and phlegm storms the pericardium and stirs liver wind, which results in convulsions of the extremities. If heat and phlegm clouds the pericardium, it results in delirium. Children born with constitutional Yin vacuity or heat retention easily suffer from heat invading the Jueyin at early stage.

Diagnosis

Diagnostic Guidelines

- Mild cases of acute onset present with fever, cough and copious phlegm in the throat. In severe cases there is shortness of breath, nasal flaring, anxiety, pale face, purple lips, and cold extremities. There may also be high fever, delirium and convulsions. Newborns and patients with a constitutional yang vacuity will present with atypical symptoms, such as no cough, high fever and shortness of breath
- Fixed rales in the lungs can be auscultated
- Chest X-ray shows flaky and patchy shadows, or uneven masses of shadows in the lungs
- CBC will help diagnose pneumonia, for example, neutrophils may be elevated or decreased
- Decreased neutrophil levels indicate a viral infection

Diagnostic Differential

- *Cough-* this may present with a fever, but there will not be shortness of breath or nasal flaring. There may be unfixed rales in the lungs.
- *Asthma-* this will present with cough and wheezing, gurgling sound in the throat, longer exhalation than inhalation and

it will re-occur. Most of the time there will be no fever. On auscultation you will hear more wheezing than rales.

Diagnostic Notes

- The relationship between the age of the child and the severity of the symptoms of Fei Yan Chuan should be considered.
- The severity of symptoms and signs, such as fever, cough, shortness of breath, nasal flaring and previous treatments should be inquired about and observed carefully.
- Carefully observe the child's following signs: spirit, respiratory rate, heart rate, pulmonary signs, index vein, color of lips and nails, fontanel development, and palpate the liver for hepatomegaly. Pay particular attention to the respiratory rate and rhythm in infants.
- CBC, chest X-ray, phlegm culture and ABG interpretation can be considered.

Pattern Differentiation

Guidelines of Differentiation

Differentiate between the common syndromes and the complicated syndromes. The main points in making this determination are the respiratory rate and rhythm, heart rate and rhythm, color of the lips, size of liver and whether or not there are convulsions and/or coma.

Differentiate between severe heat or severe phlegm. To distinguish between them, consider the severity of the fever, the presence of gurgling in the throat and shortness of breath.

Therapeutic Principle

The basic principle is to disperse and downbear the lung qi. If your pattern differentiation is wind-heat obstructing the lung, add acrid and cool herbs to clear heat. If the pattern is repletion heat and toxin stagnating in the lungs, add medicinals to expel phlegm and descend the lung qi. If the patient has a thick and greasy tongue coating, add herbs to drain dampness and clear heat. If there is blood stasis, then add herbs to regulate qi and quicken the blood. If the disease is chronic and includes qi and yin vacuity, then supplement qi and nourish yin. Supplementing qi will help to expel pathogenic factors. If there are complications, expand your pattern differentiation to include all systems involved and treat accordingly.

Patterns and treatment

Common Syndrome

Wind-heat obstructing the lung

Manifestations

Fever greater than chills, cough, shortness of breath, nasal flaring, runny nose, reddish and sore throat, red tongue with thin white or yellow coating, floating and rapid pulse, or purple index vein.

Treatment Principle Expel wind and clear heat, disperse and downbear the lung

Formula

Ma Xing Shi Gan Tang (Ephedra, Apricot, Licorice and Gypsum Decoction) and Yin Qiao San (Honeysuckle and Forsythia Powder).

Ma Huang (Ephedra) clears heat and ventilates the lungs, Shi Gao (Gypsum) clears heat in the lungs, Xing Ren (Apricot) descends lung qi and expels phlegm, Zhi Gan Cao (Prepared Licorice) generates fluids and harmonizes the middle. If the fever is severe, increase the dosage of Shi Gao (Gypsum) and also add Yu Xing Cao (Houttuynia Cordata), Huang Qin (Radix Scutellariae Baicalensis) and Zhi Zi (Fructus Gardeniae) to clear heat and toxin. If the patient has cough with a lot of phlegm, also add Qian Hu (Radix Peucedani), Gua Lou (Peel Fructus Trichosanthis), Tian Zhu Huang (Bambusa Textilis) to clear heat and eliminate phlegm.

If the throat is severely red and swollen, also add Niu Bang Zi (Fructus Arctii Lappae) and She Gan (Belamcanda Chinesis) to clear heat and soothe the throat.

Heat obstructing the lung

Manifestations

High fever, severe cough, shortness of breath, nasal flaring, yellow urine, constipation, irritability, thirst, red tongue with yellow coating, rapid pulse or purple index vein.

Treatment Principle Disperse and downbear the lung qi, clear heat and toxin

Formula

Ma Xing Shi Gan Tang (Ephedra, Apricot, Licorice and Gypsum Decoction) and Bai Hu Tang (White Tiger Decoction).

Ma Xing Shi Gan Tang (Ephedra, Apricot, Licorice and Gypsum Decoction) clears heat, disperses and downbears the lung qi. Shi Gao (Gypsum) in Bai Hu Tang (White Tiger Decoction) clears heat of the lungs and stomach, Zhi Mu (Rhizome anemarrhenae) clears heat and generates Yin. If heat is severe, add Huang Qin (Radix Scutellariae Baicalensis) and Zhi Zi (Fructus Gardeniae) to increase the function of clearing heat and toxin. If there is cough with copious phlegm, add Che Qian Zi (Plantago Asiatica) and Sang Bai Pi (Cortex Mori Albae Radicis). If the patient has constipation, add Da Huang (Radix Rhizoma Rhei).

Phlegm-heat obstructing the lung

Manifestations

Fever, severe cough with copious phlegm, gargling in the throat, shortness of breath, nasal flaring, chest fullness, poor appetite, red tongue with thick and yellow coating, slippery and rapid pulse or purple index vein.

Treatment Principle Clear heat, dissolve phlegm, disperse and downbear the lung qi

Formula

Ma Xing Shi Gan Tang (Ephedra, Apricot, Licorice and Gypsum Decoction) and Ting Li Da Zao Xie Fei Tang (Descurainia and Jujube Decoction to Drain the lung)
Ma Xing Shi Gan Tang (Ephedra, Apricot, Licorice and Gypsum Decoction) clears heat, disperses and downbears the lung Qi. Ting Li Da Zao Xie Fei Tang (Descurainia and Jujube Decoction to Drain the lung) drains heat, expels phlegm and fluids from the lung. If there is cough with copious phlegm and gargling in the throat, add Che Qian Zi (Plantago Asiatica) and Lai Fu Zi (Seman Raphani Sativi) to drain heat, dissolve phlegm and downbear the lung Qi. If there is abdominal fullness, poor appetite and a tongue with a yellow, greasy coating, add Wei Jing Tang (Reed Decoction) to clear heat and eliminate dampness. If the fever is severe, add Huang Qin (Radix Scutellariae Baicalensis) and Zhi Zi (Fructus Gardeniae) to clear heat and toxin.

Vital Qi vacuity with lingering pathogens

Yin vacuity of the lungs and stomach

Manifestations

Low grade fever, cough with scanty phlegm, thirst, flushed face, night sweats, red lips and tongue with scanty coating or peeled coating, thready and rapid pulse, or purple index vein

Treatment Principle Clear heat, disperse the lung, generate Yin and strengthen the stomach.

Formula

Sha Shen Mai Dong Tang (Glehnia and Ophiopogonis Decoction)

Sha Shen (Radix Adenophorae seu Glehniae), Mai Men Dong (Tuber Ophiopogonis Japonici), Yu Zhu (Rhizoma Polygonti Odorati) and Tian Hua Fen (Radix Trichosanthes) nourish Yin and moisten the lungs, Sang Ye (Folium Mori Albae) clears heat and expels phlegm, Bai Bian Dou (Dolichos Lablab), Gan Cao (Radix Glycyrrhizae Uralensis) supplement the vital Qi and harmonize the middle Jiao. If the patient has a long term low- grade fever, add Qing Hao (Sweet Wormwood), Di Gu Pi (Wolfberry Bark) and Hu huang Lian (Picrorhiza Rhizome) to clear vacuous heat. If there is chronic cough with sticky phlegm, add Xie Bai San (Purging White Powder) to generate Yin and clear lung-heat. If there is poor appetite due to stomach Yin vacuity, add Shan Zha (Frutus Crataegi) and Shi Hu (Dendrobium Stem) to generate fluids and strengthen the stomach.

Qi vacuity of the lung and spleen

Manifestations

Slight cough with a lot of phlegm, fatigue, pale complexion, spontaneous sweating, poor appetite, loose stool, pale tongue, thready pulse, or pale red index vein

Treatment Principle Strengthen spleen and generate qi, disperse lung and resolve phlegm

Formula

Ren Shen Wu Wei Zi Tang (Ginseng and Chinensis Decoction)
Ren Shen(Radix Ginseng), Fu Ling (Sclerotium poria cocos), Bai Zhu (Rhizoma atractylodis), Zhi Gan Cao (Honey-fried Radix Glycyrrhizae Uralensis) supplement the spleen and generate qi, disperse lungs and resolve phlegm. Wu Wei Zi (Fructus Schisandrae Chinensis) generates Yin and astringes the lungs. If there is cough with copious phlegm, add Ban Xia (Rhizoma Pinelliae Terntae), Chen Pi (Pericarpium Citri Reticulatae), Qian Hu (Radix Peucedani) and Gua Lou (Fructus Trichosanthis) to dry dampness, resolve phlegm and disperse the lungs. If there

is loose stool, add Shan Yao (Radix Dioscoreae Oppositae), Bai Bian Dou (Dolichos Lablab) to strengthen the spleen and stop diarrhea. If there is poor appetite and abdominal fullness, add Shan Zha (Frutus Crataegi) and Shen Qu (Massafermentata) to help digestion and harmonize the stomach. If there is susceptibility to cold, add Huang Qi (Radix Astragali Membranaceus), Fang Feng (Redix Ledebouriella Divaricatae) and Fu Xiao Mai (Semen Tritici Aestivi Levis) to supplement Vital and Defensive qi.

Complications

Vacuity and exhaustion of heat yang

Manifestations

Sudden onset shortness of breath, palpitations, irritability, pale complexion, purple lips, cold extremities, hepatomegaly, pale and purple tongue with white coating, deep and swift pulse or purple index vein that reaches the qi or Ming(life) gate.

Treatment Principle Restore the yang, aggressively supplement qi, rescue qi from collapse due to devastated yang

Formula

Shen Fu Long Mu Jiu Ni Tang (Gingseng, Prepared Aconite, Os Draconis and Concha Ostreae Decoction for Restoring and Reviving the yang)

Ren Shen (Radix Ginseng) aggressively supplements Yuan Qi. Zhi Fu Zi (prepared aconite) restores and revives Yang. Long Gu (Os Draconis) and Mu Li (Concha Ostreae) for stop sweating and revive Yang. Bai Shao (Radix Paeoniae Lactiflorae) and Gan Cao (Licorice Root) harmonize Ying and Wei. A patient who has the syndrome of phlegm-heat obstructing the lungs also has the symptoms of Heart qi vacuity, such as tachypnea, tachycardia, purple lips, cold extremities. The treatment strategy must include supplementing Vital qi and expelling pathogens. You may add Ren Shen (Radix Ginseng) to supplement heart qi. If the patient also has both qi and Yin vacuity of the heart; including red lips, tongue with glossy coating, add Sheng Mai San (Generate the Pulse Powder) to nourish Yin and supplement qi. If the patient also has purple lips, also add Ren Shen (Radix Ginseng), Hong Hua (Flos Carthami Tinctorii) and Ting Li Zi (Lepidium Apetalum) to supplement qi, eliminate phlegm and stop shortness of breath.

Heat invading Jueyin

Manifestations

High fever, convulsion of extremities, delirium or coma, stiff neck, blank stare, red tongue, rapid pulse, or purple index vein that reaches the Qi or Ming(life) gate.

Treatment Principle Clear heat, purge fire, calm the liver and extinguish wind.

Formula

Ling Jiao Gou Teng Tang (Antelope Horn and Uncaria Decoction) and Niu Huang Qing Xin Wan (Cattle Gallstone Pill to Clear the Heart)
    Ling Yang Jiao (Antelope Horn and Gou Teng (Ramulus Cum Uncis Uncariae) calm the liver and extinguishing wind. Fu Ling (Sclerotium poria cocos) calms the spirit and mind. Bai Shao (Radix Paeoniae Lactiflorae), Sheng Di Huang (Radix Rehmanniae Glutinosae) and Gan Cao (Radix Glycyrrhizae Uralensis) nourish Yin and relax spasms. Niu Huang Qing Xin Wan (Cattle Gallstone Pill to Clear the Heart) clears heat and purges fire. If there is high fever, add Shi Gao (Gypsum), Huang Qin (Radix Scutellariae Baicalensis) and Zhi Zi (Fructus Gardeniae) to clear heat and toxin. If the patient has convulsion of extremities, add Chan Tui (Periostracum Cicadae), Jiang Can (Bombyx Batryticatus) and Quan Xie (Buthus Martensi) to extinguish wind and stop convulsions. If there is high fever with coma and delirium, add Zi Xue Dan (Purple Snow Pill). If the patient is in a coma and there is copious phlegm in throat, add Dan Nan Xing (Prepared Arisaema

Consanguineum with gall bladder), Yu Jin (Tuber Curcumae) and Tian Zhu Huang (Concretio Silicea Bambusae) to resolve phlegm and open the orifice.

Emergency Treatment

- Exhaustion of Heart Yang: Refer to Chapter Nine, The treatment of acute cardiac insufficiency.
- Heat invading Jueyin: Refer to Chapter Nine, Emergency treatment of high fever and convulsion.

Prevention and care

- Keep the room clean with good air circulation.
- Keep the bedroom quiet, adjust the child's sleeping position regularly, pat the child's back, and if necessary, suction phlegm.
- It is appropriate to give the child liquids. You can feed them a semi-liquid diet or light and nutritious food if the child has a fever. Avoid greasy and spicy foods, dairy, these will generate heat and phlegm.

Asthma (Xiao Chuan 哮喘)

Asthma or Xiao Chuan, is a chronic lung disease that inflames and narrows the airways. It causes recurring periods of wheezing, a whistling sound when breathing, chest tightness, shortness of breath, coughing, and the need to sit upright to breathe. Most of these symptoms often occur at night or early in the morning. Zhang Zhongjing in the Han dynasty states in *Jin Kui Yao Lue* (Golden Chamber) states: "when there is a cough with shortness of breath, gargling and wheezing in the throat, use the formula is She Gan Ma Huang Tang". Xiao Chuan was first named by Zhu Danxi in the Yuan dynasty, his book *Danxi Xin Fa* (Danxi's Experiental Therapy) 1481 says: "Xiao Chuan (asthma) is primarily due to phlegm", he advocated mainly purging the pathogens during the attack stage, and mainly supplementing during the remission stage. Asthma affects people of all ages, but it most often starts during childhood, especially from 1 to 6 years old. After active treatment, many children will outgrow the disease. Some suffer with it their entire life. A chronic version is more likely to develop in children who are not treated in a timely manner, who suffer repeated attacks, who have weak constitutions or were treated incorrectly.

Etiology and Pathology

Children's asthma is caused by triggers stirring latent phlegm. The latent phlegm results from constitutional insufficiency of the lung, spleen and kidney. The triggers are exterior pathogens, allergens, emotional disorders and over exertion. The main causes are the latent phlegm resulting from constitutional insufficiency of the lung, spleen and kidney. Latent phlegm hiding inside of the body is due to abnormal water metabolism, which closely relates to the lung, spleen and kidney. Normal water metabolism relies on the lung function of dispersing and downbearing, the spleen's function of transporting and transformation, and the kidney function of warming and steaming. Children's constitutions are physiologically vulnerable, their delicate lung fail to normally disperse body fluids, therefore it remains in the lung and becomes phlegm. Their weak spleen fails to transport and transform the food, causing damp accumulation and phlegm retention. The child's kidney can't robustly warm and steam the body fluids. Moreover, the weakness of kidney yang fails to warm the spleen, leading to water retention that transforms into phlegm. Therefore, the constitutional weakness of the lung, spleen and kidney cause disorders of water metabolism leading to water retention, which in turn, transforms into latent phlegm, resulting in asthma.

Triggers

Examples of triggers are exterior pathogens, allergens, emotional disorders and over exertion.

Because children aren't likely to change their clothes with a sudden change of weather, exterior pathogens may easily invade the lungs. The lung qi fails to upbear and downbear, and the rebellious qi lingers with latent phlegm. Excessive intake of greasy, sweet, sour, salty and spicy foods, exposure to allergens (pollen, dust, paint, dander, pollution etc.) stimulate the airway and triggers the latent phlegm, inducing asthma. Emotional disorders, the liver failing course and discharge, or over exertion all cause disorders of qi and induce asthma.

Pathogenesis

Any of these mechanisms may trigger the latent phlegm. The phlegm and rebellious qi stagnate together, obstructing the airway, and result in asthma, This is manifested by periods of wheezing, a whistling sound when breathing, chest tightness, shortness of breath and cough. If the phlegm and rebellious qi are severe, blood circulation is disrupted. This disruption in the normal flow of qi and blood leads to blood stasis in the lungs and heart manifesting as a pale face, purple lips, palpitations and cold extremities due to heart yang exhaustion.

In summary, the interior cause of asthma is a constitutional vulnerability that can lead to weakness of the lung, spleen and kidney. This can cause a breakdown in water metabolism generating latent phlegm that lingers in the lung. When triggers are present, the latent phlegm and rebellious q i stagnate and obstruct the airway causing recurrent periods of wheezing. Because latent phlegm in the lung is difficult to expel, allergens can be difficult to identify, external pathogens aren't easy to avoid, and the children's lung, spleen and kidney are fragile, asthma in not an easily cured disease.

Diagnosis

Diagnostic Guidelines

- sudden onset with wheezing sound in the throat, shortness of breath, prolonged exhalation, open-mouth breathing, aiding the breathing by raising shoulders, difficult breathing when lying down.

- there are obvious triggers like sudden temperature changes or known allergens
- the child has a history of eczema or family history of asthma
- upon auscultation of the lungs there is wheezing, rales and prolonged exhalation

Diagnostic Notes

Obtain a detailed personal and family history. Clearly understand if there is a history of eczema, allergies and asthma. Try to get all of the information you can about the triggers of their asthma attacks, and all accompanying symptoms including chest tightness, fever, cough, phlegm and palpitations. Ask about the previous treatments, natures of previous episodes and response to the medicine. Pay attention to the sound, rate and rhythm of their breathing.

Refer to the blood count, chest X-ray, pulmonary function test, allergy skin test, serum specific IgE test.

Pattern Differentiation

Differentiation of Syndromes

Cough

Manifestations

Cough, no wheezing sound in throat, no shortness of breath and no difficulty in breathing. There might be unfixed rales in the lung, but no wheezing rales in all areas of the lungs.

Pneumonia

Manifestations

Fever, cough, shortness of breath, nasal flaring, but no wheezing. There is fixed moist rales but not wheezing rales in the lung.

Guidelines of Differentiation

- Differentiate between the acute stage and remission stage
  If the patient has the main symptoms of asthma, it means
  they are in the acute stage. If the main symptoms are not
  present, they are in the remission stage.
- Differentiate between cold and heat during the acute stage
  To distinguish between cold and heat assess the severity of
  sound in the throat, shortness of breath, color of face, lips,
  throat, and the tongue; consider pulse, bowel movement
  and urination as well. If it is a cold pattern there will
  be cough, shortness of breath, low-pitched wheezing,
  phlegm sounds in the throat, copious phlegm that is easy
  to expectorate, cold extremities, loose stools, pale lips and a
  tongue with a white coating. It is heat if there is cough with
  a high pitched sound in throat, coughing up yellow phlegm,
  constipation, red face, lips, throat and tongue, rapid pulse.

Differentiate the zang and fu organ systems during the
remission stage You must determine which systems are primarily
involved during the remission stage. You may see the lung, spleen
or kidney as the sole organ system involved, or you may see
multiple combinations among the three, with one or two being
dominant. During the remission stage, if there is spontaneous
sweating, recurring wheezing often aggravated by the common
cold, the pattern is lung qi vacuity. If there is a persistent cough
with phlegm, loose stool, pale complexion, then spleen qi vacuity
is the main pattern. If there is shallow breathing that is aggravated
by exertion, the complexion is pale and puffy, enuresis, profuse
nocturia, developmental delays, the pattern is kidney vacuity. If
there is spontaneous sweating, recurring wheezing often aggravated
by the common cold and loose stool, it is qi vacuity of lung and
spleen. If the patient has a lot of phlegm, loose stool, shallow
breathing aggravated by exertion, pale and puffy complexion,
enuresis, profuse nocturia, developmental delays, it is qi vacuity of
the spleen and kidney. If there is spontaneous sweating, recurring
wheezing often aggravated by the common cold, cough with
phlegm, loose stool, shallows breathing aggravated by exertion,

pale and puffy complexion, it is the vacuity of lung, spleen and kidney. The severity of these various symptoms should be assessed individually to determine which pattern is dominant. Proper assessment of root and branch mechanisms is crucial to effective treatment.

Therapeutic Principle

Acute Stage: expel phlegm, downbear the lung qi and calm wheezing. If vital qi is weak and phlegm is obstructing, then supplement qi and expel phlegm.

Remission Stage: supplement the lungs, spleen and kidney, consolidate the protective qi, supplement the spleen and expel phlegm, and supplement the kidney and grasp qi.

Patterns and treatment

Attack stage

Cold pattern of asthma

Manifestations

Cough, rapid breathing with wheezing sounds in the throat, expectoration of clear phlegm, cold extremities, loose stools, pale lips and tongue with white coating, tight and floating pulse or floating index vein.

Treatment Principle Warm the lungs, eliminate phlegm, descend Qi and calm wheezing.

Formula

Xiao Qing Long Tang (Minor Blue Green Dragon)
This formula is used for attack of wind-cold in the exterior with internal fluid-retention. In the formula, Ma Huang (Ephedra) and Gui Zhi (Cassia Twig) expel cold, disperse the lungs and

calm wheezing. Gan Jiang (Dried Ginger) warms the lungs and transforms phlegm. Bai Shao (White Peony Root) and Wu Wei Zi (Schizandra Fruit) nourish Yin and astringe the lung qi. Ban Xia (Rhizoma Pinelliae Ternae) dries damp and expels phlegm. Zhi Gan Cao (Roasted Gan Cao Licorice) supplements qi and harmonizes the middle Jiao. If the wheezing sound in the throat is severe and there is no sign of exterior cold She Gan Ma Huang Tang (Belamcanda and Ephedra Decoction) should be used. If patient has a lot clear phlegm, Su Zi (Perilla Frutescens) and Bai Jie Zi (Semen Sinapis Alae) are added to transform phlegm and calm wheezing. If cough is severe, Zi Wan (Aster Tataricus) and Kuan Dong Hua (Flos Tussilaginis Farfarae) are added to descend qi and stop cough. If there is thirst and a red tongue the pattern has transformed into heat, add Shi Gao (Gypsum) and Huang Qin (Radix Scutellariae Baicalensis) to clear interior heat.

Heat pattern of asthma

Manifestations

Rapid breathing with high pitched wheezing sounds in the throat, expectorating sticky and yellow phlegm, irritability and thirst, fever with red complexion, constipation and yellow urine, red tongue with yellow and dry coating, slippery and rapid pulse or purple and stagnating index vein.

Treatment Principle Clear the lungs, eliminate phlegm, descend Qi and calm wheezing

Formula

Ma Xing Shi Gan Tang (Ephedra, Apricot, Licorice and Gypsum Decoction).

This formula has the function of expelling evil by its pungent-cool herbs and clearing the lungs for relieving asthma due to wind heat. If there is no exterior syndrome, Ding Chuan Tang (Arrest Wheezing Decoction) can be used. If the fever is severe, increase the dosage of Shi Gao (Gypsum), and add Yu Xing Cao (Houttuynia

Cordata), Huang Qin (Radix Scutellariae Baicalensis) and Zhi Zi (Fructus Gardeniae) to clear heat and toxin. If cough is severe with phlegm, add Ting Li Zi (Lepidium Apetalum) and Che Qian Zi (Plantago Asiatica) to purge the lungs and transform phlegm. If tonsils are swollen and reddish, add Niu Bang Zi (Fructus Arctii Lappae) and She Gan (Belamcanda Chinesis) to expel toxin and soothe the throat. If the tongue coating is thick, yellow and greasy, which indicates that damp heat is severe, also add Shang Jiao Xuan Bi Tang (Dispersing Obstruction of the Upper Jiao Decoction) to disperse the lung qi and drain dampness.

Vital Qi vacuity and phlegm obstructing

Manifestations

Chronic rapid breathing that is difficult to heal, shallow breathing aggravated by exertion, wheezing sounds in throat, pale complexion, fatigue, pale lips and tongue, white coating or red tongue with yellow coating, thin pulse or index vein at qi or Ming gates.

Treatment Principle Transform phlegm, descend Qi, astringe Qi and calm wheezing.

Formula

She Gan Ma Huang Tang (Belamcanda and Ephedra Decoction) and Du Qi Wan (Capital Qi Pill).
   She Gan(Belamcanda Chinesis) and Ma Huang (Ephedra) in She Gan Ma Huang Tang (Belamcanda and Ephedra Decoction) disperse the lungs and transform phlegm, calm wheezing and soothe the throat. Gan Jiang (Rhizoma Zingiberis) Xi Xin (Herba Cun Radicae Asari) and Ban Xia (Rhizoma Pinelliae
   Terntae) warm and downbear the lung, and transform phlegm. Zi Wan (Aster Tataricus), Kuan Dong Hua (Flos Tussilaginis Farfarae) and Gan Cao (Radix Glycyrrhizae Uralensis) transform phlegm and stop cough. Wu Wei Zi (Fructus Schisandrae Chinensis) astringes the lungs and stops cough. Da Zao (Jujube) harmonizes the middle. Du Qi Wan (Capital Qi Pill) supplements

the kidney and aids the grasping of Qi. If there is cough and wheezing with lot of sweating increase the dosage of Wu Wei Zi (Fructus Schisandrae Chinensis) to astiringe the lungs and calm wheezing. If the tongue is red with a yellow coating, add Di Gu Pi (Cortex Lycii Radicis) and Mai Men Dong (Ophiopogon Root) to nourish Yin and transform phlegm. If the patient also has exhaustion of Yang, such as wheezing with rising shoulders as they breathe, pale and purple complexion, cold extremities with severe sweating, add Ren Shen (Radix Ginseng), Long Gu (Os Draconis) and Mu Li (Concha Ostreae) to strengthen Qi and revive the yang.

Remission Stage

Lung qi vacuity

Manifestations

pale complexion, spontaneous sweating, reoccurring asthma after repeated colds, fatigue, pale tongue with thin coating, thin and weak pulse or deep and pale index vein.

Treatment Principle Strengthen the lung and consolidate the exterior

Formula

Yu Ping Feng San (Jade Windscreen Powder)
In this formula, Huang Qi (Radix Astragali Membranaceus) supplements qi and consolidates the exterior. Bai Zhu (Rhizoma Atractylodis) supplements the spleen q. Fang Feng (Redix Ledebouriella divaricatae) expels wind and assists Huang Qi (Radix astragali membranaceus). If the patient is easy to sweat, add Fu Xiao Mai (Semen Tritici Aestivi Levis), Long Gu (Os Draconis) and Mu Li (Concha Ostreae) to stop sweating. If there is aversion to wind, add Gui Zhi (Cassia Twig), Bai Shao (Radix Paeoniae Lactiflorae), Sheng Jiang (Rhizoma Zingiberis Recens) and Da zao (Fructus Zizypy Jujubae) to harmonize Ying and Wei. If there is cough with a red tongue and scanty coating due to lung Yin vacuity, add Sha Shen (Radix Adenophorae Strictae) Mai

Men Dong (Tuber Ophiopogonis Japonici),Wu Wei Zi (Fructus Schisandrae Chinensis) and Bai Xian Pi (Cortex Dictammi Dasycarpi) to generate Yin and nouish the lungs.

Spleen vacuity

Manifestations

mild cough with copious phlegm, fatigue, poor appetite, loose stool, pale complexion, pale lips and tongue, thready pulse or purple index vein.

Treatment Principle Strengthen spleen and transform phlegm.

Formula

Liu Jun Zi Tang (Six Gentle Man Decoction)
   In this formula, Si Jun Zi Tang (Four Gentle Man Decoction) supplements the spleen qi. Chen Pi (Pericarpium Citri Reticulatae) and Ban Xia (Rhizoma Pinelliae Terntae) dry dampness and transform phlegm. If there is poor appetite, add Shan Zha (Frutus Crataegi), Mu Gua (Chaenomeles Lagenaria) to transform stomach and aid digestion. If there is cough with a lot phlegm, add Su Zi (Perilla Frutescens) and Bai Jie Zi (Semen Sinapis Alae) to transform phlegm and downbear qi. If there is loose stool, add Shan Yao (Radix Dioscoreae Oppositae), Bai Bian Dou (Dolichos Lablab) to supplement spleen and stop diarrhea.

Kidney vacuity

Manifestations

Cold extremities, shallow breathing aggravated by exertion, soreness and weakness of the low back and knees, profuse nocturia or enuresis, developmental delays, pale complexion, pale lips and tongue or red tongue with scanty coating, thready pulse or deep index vein.

Treatment Principle Supplement the kidney and grasp qi

Formula

Jin Gui Shen Qi Wan (Kidney Qi Pill from the Golden Cabinet)

In this formula, Zhi Fu Zi (Prepared Aconite) and Rou Gui (Cortex Cinnamomi Cassiae) warm kidney yang, Liu Wei Di Huang Wan (Six-ingredient Pill with Rehmannia) nourishes and supplements the kidney. If there are severe signs of kidney Yin vacuity, such as slim body, red tongue with scanty coating, take out of Zhi Fu Zi (Prepared Aconite) and Rou Gui (Cortex Cinnamomi Cassiae), and add Mai Men Dong (Tuber Ophiopogonis Japonici),Wu Wei Zi (Fructus Schisandrae Chinensis) to enrich the kidney Yin and grasping qi function. If there is profuse nocturia add Wu Yao (Radix Linderae) and Yi Zhi Ren (Fructus Aliniae Oxyphyllae) to consolidate the kidney and control urine. If both kidney yin and yang are vacuous, then use Shen Ge San (Radix Ginseng and Gecko Powder) and add Yin Yang Huo (Herba Epinedii) and Wu Wei Zi (Fructus Schisandrae Chinensis) to supplement kidney yin and yang. If there is dual vacuity of the lung and kidney, add Jin Shui Liu Jun Jian (Six-Gentleman of Metal and Water Decoction) to enrich kidney yin, supplement spleen and transform phlegm.

Prevention and care

- dress the child in layers or bring extra clothes to meet the demands of changing weather. This will minimize over exposure to cold. If they are treated in time, they will probably only show signs of the exterior pattern.
- Avoid contact with allergens such as pollen, dust, paint, shellfish etc.
- Reduce hyperactivity and emotional distress
- Focus on the remission stage to prevent asthma attacks
- The child's bedroom should have good air circulation and plenty of sunshine if possible. If the climate is frequently cloudy, full spectrum lighting should be considered. The room's temperature should be comfortable and stable as seasons change.
- Ideally, the house should have hard flooring, not carpet.

Diseases and Syndromes of the Spleen and Stomach

The diseases and syndromes of the spleen and stomach systems are mainly located in the spleen and stomach. The spleen and stomach are localized in the middle Jiao and belong to the earth phase. The spleen belongs to yin earth, it likes dryness and dislikes moisture. The spleen governs the transporting and transforming of food, which depends on the ascending function of the spleen. So it is said that spleen is in the normal condition if it can ascend. The spleen produces the qi and blood and ascends the clear qi and nourishing the whole body. It is the acquired foundation and the source of qi and blood. The spleen has the function of controlling blood, dominating the extremities and the muscles. It opens into the mouth and has its outward manifestation on the lips. The stomach belongs to Yang earth. It likes moisture and dislikes dryness. The stomach governs receiving and digesting of food. It is the sea of food which depends on the descending function of stomach. So it is said that the stomach is harmonious when it can descend.

There is an exterior and interior relationship between the spleen and stomach. They cooperate to complete the function of receiving, digesting, transporting and transforming. Only with the ascending of the spleen and descending of the stomach and the balance between dryness and moisture of spleen and stomach, can the spleen transport and stomach receive food normally. Thus, all disorders of the spleen and stomach come from disharmony between dryness and moisture, ascending and descending of the spleen and stomach. Imbalances may result in improper production of qi and blood affecting the other organs.

Based on this understanding, the main therapies are:

- harmonize the dryness and moisture of the spleen and stomach
- regulate the ascending and descending function of the spleen and stomach
- strengthen the transporting and transformation of spleen and stomach.

The child's spleen tend to be vulnerable, their stomachs are smaller and cannot contain a large amounts of food. It is common for children to have disorders of the spleen and stomach. It doesn't only affect the production of qi and blood, it may also result in slow development. Therefore, it is key for children's development to regulate the function of the spleen and stomach. This, in turn, regulates the ascending, descending, dryness and moisture of the spleen and stomach. Moderate therapies are utilized to avoid the use of strong purging and supplementing methods. Manual therapies such as Tui Na and diet should be widely used for disorders of the spleen and stomach in pediatrics.

Oral Thrush (E Kou Chuang 鹅口疮)

E in Chinese means goose, Kou means mouth, and Chuang means sores. E Kou Chuang (oral thrush) means whitish patches and sores in the mouth that looks like the mouth of a goose. Oral thrush is whitish patches on the lips, tongue, or inside the cheeks that look a little like pieces of cottage cheese but can't be wiped away. Scraping the white patches off can cause some bleeding. Oral thrush can affect anyone, but infants of low birth weight and premature babies have higher incidence. Many babies don't feel anything at all, but some may be uncomfortable when sucking. Some babies may not feed well because their mouth feels sore. Oral thrush was recorded first in the Sui dynasty. *In the Zhu Bing Yuan Huo Lun* (General Treatise on the Causes and symptoms of diseases) byChao Yuan-fang in 610 it states "whitish patches or sores on the tongue, and insides of the cheeks look like the mouth of a goose. It is oral thrush." Until the Ming dynasty, a physician, Chen Shi Gong pointed out the cause, manifestation, and therapy of oral thrush. He said in *Wai Ke Zheng Zong* (Orthodox Manual of Surgery) 1617 "Oral thrush is due to the spleen and heart being invaded by fetus heat, which is manifested with whitish patches likes snow all over the mouth, forming in piles with swelling, resulting in difficulty sucking and crying, ... put Bing Peng San (Borneol and Borax Powder) externally and locally while orally taking Liang Ge San (Cool the Diaphragm Powder)".

Etiology and Pathology

Oral thrush is mainly caused by heat accumulating in the mouth with turbid toxin invading the mouth. It is divided into a repletion type that is the heat accumulation of spleen and heart, and vacuity type that is vacuous fire stirring up due to congenital vacuity or chronic diseases

Heat accumulation of the spleen and heart

The pregnant woman has heat accumulation of the spleen and heart due to their preference of pungent, spicy and fried foods during pregnancy, which results in heat accumulation of the spleen and heart, and then transfers to the fetus. In addition, a newborn mouth is not washed cleanly, and easily suffers from turbid toxin, which stagnates in the spleen and heart transforming into fire. Since the spleen opens into the mouth and the tongue is the sprout of the heart, the heat stirs up in the mouth and tongue and results in whitish patches in the whole mouth.

Hyperactivity of vacuous fire

This is due to congenital vacuity, prolonged vomiting and diarrhea, and improper feeding impairing body fluids. Therefore fire is not able to be controlled by water, vacuous fire then flames upwards resulting in whitish patches in the mouth.

Diagnosis

Diagnostic Guidelines

- The whitish patches may be on the tongue, cheek, gum, palate, and even spreading to the throat. It may affect feeding and breathing.
- It usually occurs in newborn and weak children who have prolonged illness, or are treated by antibiotics for long courses.
- Candida albicans and its spores can be found in the whitish patches when checked by microscope.

Differential Diagnosis

- Mouth ulcers can occur in infants, toddlers, and young children. They are pale, yellowish or whitish ulcers on the tongue mucosa that are surrounded by redness. There is also a local burning pain.
- Diphtheria is an acute infectious disease caused by the bacteria *Corynebacterium diphtheriae*. There will be fever, cough and possibly a gray there may be a gray to black covering (pseudomembrane) in the throat, enlarged lymph glands and swelling of the neck or larynx. It is a critical disease.

Diagnostic Notes

- The children's mouth should be carefully observed. If there are whitish crumbs on the tongue and mouth, it should be considered as thrush.
- The whitish crumbs can be gently wiped with cotton swab to be checked by microscope to confirm diagnosis.
- The child's age should be considered, or if any improper feeding history exists. If there was any long-term history of taking antibiotics as well as oral hygiene history should be inquired about.

Pattern Differentiation

Guidelines for differentiation

Differentiating between repletion and vacuity is the primary criteria. If it is acute with a short history of the disease, a lot of whitish patches in the mouth that are surrounded by redness with thirst, pain, and fever. It is a repletion pattern. If it is chronic with only mild whitish patches in the mouth with no surrounding redness, and accompanied with symptoms of spleen and heart vacuity. It is a vacuity pattern.

Therapeutic Principle

The main therapy for replete heat patterns is to clear heat, eliminate toxin and purge fire. For vacuity patterns you must for nourish yin, descend fire and calm yang.

Patterns and treatment

Heat accumulation of the spleen and heart

Manifestations

Several whitish patches in the mouth that are surrounded by redness, thirst, anxiety, crying with no sucking, fever, constipation, yellow urine, red tongue with thick and yellow greasy tongue coating. Index vein is purple and stagnated, slippery and rapid pulse.

Treatment Principle Clear the heart and purge the spleen

Formula

Qing Re Xie Pi San (Clear heat and purge the spleen powder)
In the formula, Huang Lian (rhizoma coptidis) and Zhi Zi (Fructus Gardeniae Jasminoidis) clear the heart and purging heat. Huang Qin (Radix scutellariae baicalensis) and Shi Gao (Gypsum)

spread the accumulation of heat of the spleen. Sheng Di Huang (Radix Rehmanniae Glutinosae) clears heat and cools blood. Deng Xin Cao (Juncos Effusus) clears heat, descends fire, and guides heat downward. If there is constipation, add Da Huang (Radix et Rhizoma Rhei) to purge heat from the Fu organs. If thirsty and drinking water a lot, also add Shi Hu (Dendrobium Stem) and Yu Zhu (Rhizoma Polygonti Odorati) to nourish Yin and generating fluid.

Vacuous fire flaring upward

Manifestations

Scattered whitish patches in the mouth, surrounded by redness that is not obvious, weak constitution, pale complexion with red cheek, low grade fever, loose stool, no thirst, tender and red tongue with a scanty coating, pale index vein, thready pulse.

Treatment Principle Nourish yin and descend fire

Formula

Zhi Bai Di Huang Wan (Anemarrhena, Phellodendron, and Rehmannia pill)
    In the formula, Shu Di Huang (Radix Rehmanniae Glutinosae Conquitae) nourishes the kidney essence, Ze Xie (Alisma Plantago-aquatica) eliminates dampness in the lower Jiao, Shan Zhu Yu (Fructus Corni Officinalis) supplements the liver and kidney, Mu Dan Pi (Cortex Moutan Radicis) clears liver fire, Shan Yao (Radix Dioscoreae Oppositae) and Fu Ling (Sclerotium Poria Cocos) strengthens the spleen and eliminates dampness, Zhi Mu (Rhizome Anemarrhenae) and Huang Bai (Cotex Phellodendri) nourish Yin and descend fire. If the spleen Qi is weak, add. Huang Qi (Radix Astragali Membranaceus). If the vacuous fire is flaring upward due to fire not being controlled by water, add Rou Gui (Cortex Cinnamomi Cassiae). If there is Yin vacuity, add Sha Shen (Radix Adenophorae Strictae), Mai Men Dong (Tuber Ophiopogonis Japonici) and Yu Zhu (Rhizoma Polygonti Odorati)

Other Treatment

- Patent herbs Dao Chi San (Guide Red Powder) Taken orally 0.1~0.25g for per time, 3 times per day. It is used for heat retention in the heart and spleen.
- Tui Na Clearing the spleen and stomach, clearing Tian He Shui. If there is fever, add clearing six Fu organs technique. If there are palpitations and anxiety, add Tui Xiao Tian Xin.
- Topical therapy
- Bing Peng San (Borneol and Borax Powder) place locally, 3 times/day. This is used for repletion heat pattern.
- Wu Yu Gao(Evodia Ointment) Wu Zhu Yu (Fructus Evodia Rutaecapae)10g is mixed with vinegar as a paste and put it on Ki1, once per day. Used for vacuous fire.

Prevention and care

- Nursing mothers should try to avoid excess pungent, hot, dry and greasy food
- Strongly recommend breastfeeding. Then add foods in a timely and reasonable way
- Pay close attention to the child's oral hygiene, regularly disinfect the feeding bottles, and pacifiers to prevent them from contamination
- Try to avoid long-term treatment with antibiotics, especially for children who have chronic diarrhea and vomiting
- Frequently give water to ill children, and avoid feeding them too much hot, hard and spicy food

Aphtha (Kou Chuang 口疮)

Aphtha refers to small ulcers in the oral mucous membranes that are painful, covered by a gray exudate, surrounded by an erythematous halo. If the ulcers are larger, even erosion in the whole mouth, it is called mouth erosion (Kou Mi). If the ulcers are at the corners of mouth, it is Yan Kou Chuang (aphtha like a mouth of a swallow). Patients of all ages may suffer from this disease, but the incidence is much higher in infants. It can appear in any season. Aphtha was first recorded in the *Huang Di Nei Jing Su Wen* on aphtha(Yellow Emperor Classic of TCM. Movement of qi) it states "The movement of metal is in balance, the qi movement of fire and wood will be respectively hyperactive therefore aphtha occurs." It is pointed out that the aphtha is related to heat evils. Chao Yuan Fang in his book, *Zhu Bing Yuan Huo Lun* (General Treatise on the Causes and symptoms of diseases) 610 stated: "Pediatric aphtha is due to yang hyperactivity and feeding too hot, which leads to heat in the heart flaring upward, resulting in aphtha. " It says that aphtha is due to excessive heat in the heart. *Xiao Er Wei Sheng Zhong Wei Fanh Lun* (General Treatise on hygiene in Children) 1156 stated: "Wind, toxin, dampness and heat along with the accumulation of qi and blood will invade at weak points, which causes sores. If the sores occur on the lips and inside of the cheeks, it is aphtha. If it occurs in the corners of lips, it is Yan Kou aphtha. Stomatitis and angular stomatitis in western medicine correlates to the category of aphtha.

Etiology and Pathology

The major cause of this disease is due to the invasion of the exterior evils, wind-heat lodged in the spleen, or accumulated heat in the heart and spleen, or a weak constitution allowing flaring of vacuous fire.

Invading of the exterior evils

After wind-heat invades the body through the skin and muscles, it affects the spleen and stomach interiorly. Because the heart opens at the tongue and the tongue is the sprout of the heart, the wind-heat stirs upward with toxin and disturbs the heart and spleen, this heat in the mucosal membranes results in aphtha.

Heat accumulating in the heart and spleen

Incorrect nursing and feeding, such as overfeeding of greasy, sweet, fried and spicy foods all produce heat interiorly, which accumulates in the heart and spleen resulting in aphtha.

After a prolonged illness, such as chronic vomiting, diarrhea, or a weak constitution results the consumption of Yin fluid. Water then fails to control fire, the fire flares upward, thus causing ulcerations.

Diagnosis

Diagnostic Guidelines

There are ulcers on the tongue or cheek, gum and palate, which may even be erosion, salivation, and pain. If it is due to exogenous pathogens, it may be associated with fever and the enlargement of the submandibular lymph nodes.

Differential Diagnosis

Oral thrush It likely occurs in newborns or infants who are younger than 1 year old, and it is manifested by whitish patches on the lips, tongue, or inside the cheeks that look a little like cottage cheese.

Diagnostic Notes

- Pay attention if there are ulcers and erosions on the tongue, cheek, gum and palate
- Ask the history of the disease, which relates to the medicine the patients are taking, such as antibacterial, steroid
- Inquire about the history of nursing and feeding
- It is necessary to check the blood count if the patient has a fever

Pattern Differentiation

Guidelines of differentiation

Differentiate between repletion and vacuity

If the onset is acute, has a short history of the disease, and the ulcers are severe and painful, or accompanied with fever, it belongs to repletion. If it is chronic, there is long term history of the disease, and only mild ulcers. It belongs to vacuity pattern.

Differentiate between the zang and fu

If there are more ulcers on the tongue or cheek, gum and palate, it likely belongs to disorders of the spleen and stomach. If there are more ulcers on the tip or sides of tongue, it likely belongs to the heart.

Therapeutic Principle

For the repletion heat pattern, clear heat, eliminate toxin and purge the heat from the spleen and heart. For vacuity pattern, nourish Yin, descend fire and guide the yang back to the Mingmen.

Patterns and treatment

Wind-heat invading the spleen

Manifestations

The ulcers are on the tongue, cheek, gum and palate, and they are surrounded by redness. The patient refuses to eat due to the local pain, crying with anxiety, foul smelling breath, salivation, yellow urine, constipation, fever, red tongue with yellow coating, floating and rapid pulse, or floating and purple index vein.

Treatment principle Expel wind, clear heat and toxin

Formula

Liang Ge San (Cooling Diaphragm Powder)
    In the formula, Huang Qin (Radix Scutellariae Baicalensis), Zhi Zi (Fructus Gardeniae) and Lian Qiao (Fructus Forsythiae Suspensae) clear heat and resolve toxin. Da Huang (Radix et Rhizoma Rhei) and Mang Xiao (Mirabilitum) promote the Fu and purge fire. Dan Zhu Ye (Herba Lophatheri) clears heat and relieves anxiety, Gan

Cao (Radix Glycyrrhizae Uralensis) and Bo He (Herba Menthae Haplocalycis) resolve stagnated heat and toxin. If the patient has fever, add Chai Hu (Radix Bupleuri) and Shi Gao (Gypsum).

Heat accumulation in the spleen and stomach

Manifestations

There are ulcers and a lot of erosion are on the tongue, cheek, gum and palate that is surrounded by redness, severe local pain, anxiety, thirsty, salivation, yellow urine with constipation, fever, red tongue with yellow coating, drinking a lot water, red tongue with yellow coating, slippery and rapid pulse or deep, purple and stagnated index vein.

Treatment Principle Clear and purge the heat of heart and spleen.

Formula

Dao Chi San (Guide Red Powder) and Xie Huang San (Purge Yellow Powder).

In the formula, Zhi Zi (Fructus Gardeniae Jasminoidis), Huang Lian (Rhizoma Coptidis) and Dan Zhu Ye (Herba Lophatheri) clear heart heat, Sheng Di Huang (Radix Rehmanniae Glutinosae) cools the blood. Tong Cao (Tetrapanax Papyriferus) guides heat downward. Fang Feng (Radix Saposhnikoviae) and Shi Gao (Gypsum) resolve the stagnated heat in the spleen. If the patient has scanty urine, add Che Qian Zi (Plantago Asiatica), Hua Shi (Talcum) to promote urination and to clear heat. If the patient has thirst, add Tian Hua Fen (Radix Trichosanthis) to clear heat and generate fluids.

Flaring of vacuous fire

Manifestations

Ulcers in the mouth that are surrounded by only mild redness, mild pain, chronic and long term, fatigue, thirst, red tongue with scanty coating or peeled coating

Treatment Principle

Nourish yin, descend fire and guide yang to the Mingmen

Formula

Liu Wei Di Huang Wan(Six-ingredient Pill with Rehmannia)
   In the formula, Shu Di Huang (Radix Rehmanniae Glutinosae Conquitae) and Ze Xie (Alisma Plantago-aquatica) supplement the kidney and clear heat. Shan Zhu Yu (Fructus Corni Officinalis) and Mu Dan Pi (Cortex Moutan Radicis) supplement the liver and clear heat. Shan Yao (Radix Dioscoreae Oppositae) and Fu Ling (Sclerotium Poria Cocos) transform the spleen and eliminate dampness. Add Rou Gui (Cortex Cinnamomi Cassiae) to guide Yang to the Mingmen.

Other Treatment

Patent herbs

- Huang Lian Jie Du Pian (Coptis Detoxicating Pills), Taken orally 1~2 pill per time, 3 times per day. It is used for aphtha due to excessive heat.
- Zhi Bai Di Huang Wan (Anemarrhena, Phellodendron, and Rehmannia Pill), taken orally 1 pill per time, 3 times per day. It is used for aphtha due to vacuity fire.

Topical therapy

- Bing Peng San (Borneol and Borax Powder) local application, 3 times/day. Used for repletion heat pattern.
- Wu Yu Gao (Evodia Ointment) Wu Zhu Yu (Fructus Evodia Rutaecapae)10g is mixed with vinegar as a paste and placed on Ki1, once per day. Used for vacuity fire.

Prevention and care

- Pay close attention to the child's oral hygiene, regularly disinfect the feeding bottles
- Try to avoid too much pungent, hot, dry and greasy food

Vomiting (Ou Tu 呕 吐)

Vomiting is a symptom of the spleen and stomach. It is a very common clinical disorder of this system. Vomiting was first documented in the *Huang Di Nei Jing*, which said "If cold evil stays in stomach and intestine, resulting in the qi adversely moving upward it leads to vomiting." Chapter 74 of the *Huang Di Nei Jing* says: "Most of the strong vomiting that is sour along with diarrhea belongs to a heat pattern." The *Nei Jing* considers the causes of vomiting to be cold, heat and food stagnation. The location is in the stomach. The patterns of vomiting in *Xiao Er Wei Sheng Zhong Wei Fang Lun* (General hygiene of pediatrics) 1156 are due to heat, wind, food stagnation, fear, disorders of the stomach qi, vacuity cold and incorrect nursing. *You You Ji Cheng* (Collection of Pediatrics) 1750, summarizes the pathology of vomiting as the stomach qi adversely moving upward due to disorders of the stomach. Vomiting may occur at any age, but most likely occurs in newborn and infant children.

Etiology and Pathology

- Invasion of exterior pathogenic factors
- The exterior pathogen, such as warm evil directly invades the stomach Fu organ through mouth and nose, which leads to the stomach failing to descend, therefore the stomach Qi counterflows, resulting in vomiting
- Food stagnation
- All of the causes, such as incorrect care or irregular feeding lead to food stagnating in the stomach and disturbing the ascending and descending of stomach Qi. This results in counterflow of the stomach Qi, and causes vomiting
- Yang vacuity of the spleen and stomach

- If the constitution of the spleen and stomach Yang is weak, or if the children are fed too much cold food, then the cold food stagnates in the stomach and intestine, leading to vomiting due to the stomach Qi failing to descend
- Vomiting due to fear
- Children's minds are weak and their brains are undeveloped. Their Qi is disturbed easily by fear. If the Qi becomes disorderly and affects the stomach this leads to vomiting due to the failure of stomach Qi to descend resulting in vomiting

Generally, the location of this disease is primarily in the stomach, but it relates to liver and spleen as well. The causes are exterior factors, summer heat, food stagnation, the vacuity of the spleen and stomach Yang, or sudden fear. All of them lead to vomiting due to the stomach Qi failing to descend.

Diagnosis

Diagnostic Guidelines

- The main manifestation is milk or food exiting from the mouth
- There is a history of invasion by exterior pathogenic factors, food stagnation, vacuity cold of the spleen and stomach, or emotional disorders

Diagnostic Notes

- Pay attention to when the vomiting occurs, if it relates to diet, the frequency and volume of the vomitus
- Carefully ask the history of vomiting and accompanying symptoms, such as if the patient has headache, fever, convulsion and bowl movement
- Perform a thorough and careful physical examination, paying particular attention to abdominal palpation
- Inquire if the stool is unobstructed, or if there is recurring and severe vomiting. Abdominal X-ray or abdominal B-ultrasonic is necessary for severe cases

Pattern Differentiation

Guide lines of differentiation

Differentiate between exterior attack and food stagnation. If it is due to the invasion of exterior factors, the manifestations of exterior wind cold or heat will be present. If it is due to food stagnation, there is a history of overeating, unsanitary food or irregular eating; the vomiting may be accompanied with sour food and stomachache.

Differentiate between cold, heat, vacuity and repletion. If the patient has vomiting after eating, but significant time elapses between eating and vomiting, and the vomitus is clear and thin, it is due to cold. If the patient has vomiting immediately after eating, and the vomitus has a strong odor, is sour and thin, it is due to heat. If the vomitus contains undigested food and there is fatigue, it is a vacuity pattern. If the patient feels better after vomiting, it is a repletion pattern.

Therapeutic Principle

The basic therapy is to descend the stomach Qi and stop vomiting.

Differentiation of Patterns

Exterior Evils Invading the Stomach

Manifestations

Sudden vomiting, runny nose, chills and fever, loose stool, pink or pale tongue with white and greasy coating, floating pulse, reddish index vein.

Treatment principle Expel wind, release exterior, harmonize the middle and stop vomiting

Formula

Huo Xiang Zheng Qi San (Agastache Powder rectify qi)

In the formula, Huo Xiang (Agastache) eliminates dampness, regulating Qi and harmonizing the middle. Zi Su Ye (Perilla Leaf) and Bai Zhi (Dahurian Angelica Root) expels the exterior wind-cold and regulates dampness. Ban Xia (Rhizoma Pinelliae Ternae) and Chen Pi (Pericarpium Citri Reticulatae) regulate qi and resolve phlegm. Bai Zhu (Rhizoma Atractylodis Macrocephalae), Fu Ling (Sclerotium Poriae Cocos) and Zhi Gan Cao (Roasted Licorice) harmonize the middle and resolve dampness. If there is fullness of the abdomen, add Mu Xiang (Radix Aucklandiae Lappae) and Zhi Ke (Bitter Orange Peel). If there is severe abdominal pain, add Bai Shao (Radix Paeoniae Lactiflorae).

Food stagnation

Manifestations

Vomiting with undigested food or milk that has a sour odor, frequent vomiting, feels better after vomiting, thirst, crying and anxiety, refusal to eat, fullness and pain of the abdomen, red tongue with yellow and greasy coating, slippery and wiry pulse, or purple and stagnated index vein.

Treatment principle Digest the food and guide stagnated food downwards, harmonize the stomach and stop vomiting.

Formula

Bao He Wan (Harmony Preserving Pills)

In the formula, Shen Qu (Medicated Leaven) and Lai Fu Zi (Semen Raphani Sativi) promote digestion of stagnated food, resolve fullness of the abdomen, and guide the stagnated Qi and food downwards. Ban Xia (Rhizoma Pinelliae Terntae) and Chen Pi (Pericarpium Citri Reticulatae) harmonize the stomach and stop vomiting. Lian Qiao (Fructus Forsythiae Suspensae) clears stagnantion heat. If the patient has constipation, add Da Huang

(Radix et Rhizoma Rhei). If the patient has thirst, add Tian Hua Fen (Radix Trichosanthes).

Vacuity Cold of the spleen and stomach

Manifestations

Delayed vomiting after eating, which is clear, thin, no odor or contains phlegm, pale face, tired, cold extremities, dull abdominal pain, clear urine, pale tongue with white coating, thready pulse.

Treatment principle Warm the middle and expel cold

Formula

Ding Yu Li Zhong Tang (Clove and Evodia Decoction to Regulate the Middle)

In the formula, Dang Shen (Radix Codonopsitis Pilosulae), Gan Cao (Radix Glycyrrhizae) and Bai Zhu (Rhizoma Atractylodis) supplement the spleen, nourish the stomach, and fortify the middle Qi. Ding Xiang (Flos Caryophylli), Wu Zhu Yu (Fructus Evodiae Rutaecarpae) and Gan Jiang (Rhizoma Zingiberis) warm the middle, expel cold, descend the adverse Qi and stop vomiting. If there is vomiting with clear water, dull pain of the abdomen and cold extremities, add Fu Zi (Radix Aconiti Carmichaeli) and Rou Gui (Cortex Cinnamomi Cassiae).

Vomiting due to fear

Manifestations

Vomiting after falling down or being scared, pale or purple complexion, anxiety, tossing and turning, crying with screaming, wiry pulse or purple index vein.

Treatment Principle Soothe the liver, regulate qi, strengthen the spleen and calm the fear

Formula

Ding Tu Wan (Stop Vomiting Pill)
   In the formula, Quan Xie (Buthus Martensi) calms fear, Ding Xiang (Flos Caryophylli) and Ban Xia (Rhizoma Pinelliae Ternae) harmonize the stomach, descend Qi and stop vomiting. If there is dizziness, add Ju Hua (Flos Chrysanthemi Morifolii) and Tian Ma (Rhizoma Gastrodiae Elatae).

Other Treatment

Patent herbs

- Huo Xiang Zheng Qi Ye (Agastache Liquid Rectify Qi), taken orally 5ml-10ml for per time, 3 times per day. It is used for vomiting due to summer-heat and dampness.
- Xiang Sha Yang Wei Wan (Aucklandiae Lappae and Adenphorae Gleniae Strengthen Stomach), taken orally 1/2 pill-1pill for per time, 3 times per day. It is used for vomiting due to vacuity cold of the spleen and stomach.

Acupuncture therapy

- Ren12, PC6, St36, Sp4 and Ub21. If it is due to heat, add LI4. If due to cold, add Ren13, Du14. If there is food stagnation, add Ren11. If there is liver qi stagnation, add GB34 and Liv3, once per day.

Ear points

Stomach, Liver, Sympathetic, Subcortex and Shen Men. 2~3 points for each time, strong stimulation, leave the needles about 15 minutes, once per day.

Tuina

- If vomiting is due to food stagnation, do the following Tuina: kneading LI4, purging large intestine, dividing Yin and Yang, supplementing the spleen meridian, clearing the stomach, softening Banmen and St36, clearing Tian He Shui, transforming inner Bagua.

- If vomiting is due to replete heat, also use clearing the spleen, stomach and large intestine. Kneading LI4, purging six Fu, transforming inner Bagua, clearing Tian He shui, calming the liver and dividing Yin and Yang.
- If vomiting is due to vacuity cold, also use the following Tuina, supplementing spleen, softening outside Laogong, pushing Sanguan, softening Ren12, dividing Yin and Yang, transforming inner Bagua.

Topical therapy

- Slice fresh ginger as thick as 0.1~0.3cm and 1cm in diameter. Bandage it to PC6 to prevent vomiting.
- Mix Wu Zhu Yu (Fructus Evodia Rutaecapae)30g with fresh ginger 3g and green
- Onions 3g. Make it into a paste and put it on Ren8, once per day. Used for vomiting due to cold.

Prevention and care

Avoid feeding for 4~6 hours if the child has severe vomiting. Fresh ginger cooked with water or rice cooked with water is recommended. Gradually give food that is easily digested and decrease the volume of food given.

Diarrhea (Xie Xie 泄 泻)

Diarrhea is a common disorder of the spleen and stomach. It refers to increased frequency of loose stool, and in severe cases, watery feces. The diarrhea may occur in any season, but has a higher incidence in the summer and fall. The age of the highest incidence is mainly in infants and young children, 6 months to 2 years of age. Mild diarrhea has a good prognosis, but it may have complications and can be critical, such as in the case of yin and yang exhaustion syndrome due to acute and severe diarrhea, which results in damage of the Yin fluid. Another example of severe diarrhea is Gan Ji (malnutrition) or chronic convulsion due to chronic diarrhea. Therefore, pediatric diarrhea is one of the main mechanisms resulting in slow growth and development in children, and even death. Diarrhea was recorded first in *Huang Di Nei Jing· Zhi Zhun Yao Da Lun*(Yellow Emperor Classic of TCM·), it said "If the Tai Yin is excessive due to dampness, it will result in diarrhea." Diarrhea was divided into four categories; due to food stagnation, fear, cold, and heat. In *A New book of Pediatrics*, 1132, physician Wan Quan in Ming dynasty summarized four therapies of diarrhea, such as warming and transforming, lifting, dividing and astringing, he accumulated a wealth of theoretical and empirical treatment for children's diarrhea. Zhang Jing Yue in his book, *The Collected Treatises of Jing-Yue*, 1624, on diarrhea it said: "if the spleen and stomach are damaged, the water will turn into dampness, and the food will turn into stagnation". He pointed out that diarrhea was related to the spleen and stomach.

Etiology and Pathology

The main causes of diarrhea are improper diet, exterior pathogens and vacuity of the spleen and stomach.

- Improper diet
  The pediatric spleen is commonly insufficient, the stomach is small and tender and cannot contain large amounts of food. If patients are nursed and fed inappropriately, such as being allowed to overeat cold foods or eating contaminated food the spleen and stomach may become injured and impair their ability to transform and transport, resulting in the mixture with clear and turbid Qi causing diarrhea.

- Invasion of exterior pathogen
  In children the functions of the zang and fu organs are insufficient and the skin is tender. This can allow exterior pathogenic factors to easily invade. When dampness invades the body, it may disturb the spleen function and result in

diarrhea. An ancient physician said: "No dampness, no diarrhea."

- Vacuity of the spleen and stomach
  Children who are born prematurely, have an obstructed labor or low birth weight are likely to have a weak spleen and stomach function. In addition children who are fed and nursed incorrectly, will also experience vacuity of the spleen and stomach. Therefore the spleen fails to transform and transport the food, clear Qi fails to ascend, resulting in the food transforming into dampness and water, leading to diarrhea.

- Yang vacuity of the spleen and Kidney
  Yang vacuity of the spleen and Kidney is caused by chronic diarrhea, and weakness of the Mingmen fire. Yin cold becomes excessive due to the weak Yang of the spleen and kidney, which results in failure of transformation and transportation. hence the undigested food goes to large intestine and shows the diarrhea.

The children who suffer from diarrhea also easily have other complications, such as consumption of the Qi and Yin, even exhaustion of Qi and body fluid, chronic convulsions or malnutrition because children's young Yang is insufficient and their young Yin is imperfect.

In summary, the location of diarrhea is mainly in the spleen, and the main pathogen is dampness.

Diagnosis

Diagnostic Guidelines

- Increased frequency of loose stool, 3~5times a day, even more than 10 times a day. The feces is slightly yellowish, it looks like egg drops in the soup or brown with a foul odor. It may be accompanied by mucus in the stool, nausea, vomiting, abdominal pain, fever and thirst

- There is a history of incorrect feeding, eating contaminated food, or invasion by exterior evils
- Severe cases may have scanty urine, high fever, anxiety, fatigue, dry skin, sunken fontanel, orbital subsidence, crying without tears, cherry red lips, bloating

Differentiation of Diagnosis

- Physiological diarrhea It often happens in infants younger than 6 months who are obese and have eczema. The diarrhea occurs shortly after birth, but it does not affect the growth and development of the child. The stool will gradually become normal after supplementing with food.
- Dysentery The manifestations of dysentery are increased frequency of bowel movement with mucus, pus and blood, obvious tenesmus, fever. WBC and RBC are found in stool examination. Shigella can be found feces culture.

Diagnostic Notes

- Know the times, volume, texture of bowel movement and accompanying manifestations in detail
- To distinguish the severities of dehydration in children observe their complexion and spirit. Observe if the orbitals or fontanels appear sunken. Inquire about thirst, and the volume of urine.
- Ask age of children and feeding habits
- Do a laboratory exam of the feces. It is necessary to check the CBC, feces culture, carbon dioxide and electrolytes if the patient has fever,

Pattern Differentiation

Guidelines of differentiation

Differentiating between common syndromes and complicated syndromes

If a case is prolonged, and there is increased frequency of loose stool or watery feces, but there are no signs of dehydration due to qi and yin being injured, it is considered a mild case of diarrhea. If the patient has severe diarrhea with oliguria or no urine, dry skin, sunken eyes and fontanels, thirst, red and dry lips, it is a severe case.

Differentiating between the causes of diarrhea

If the diarrhea contains undigested food, pale color, and sour odor, it is due to milk stagnation. If there is loose and yellow stool with a lot of water, abdominal pain, it is due to damp-heat. If the feces is watery with light odor and foam, accompanied with paroxysmal abdominal pain, it is due to wind cold. if the feces are loose with undigested food, the diarrhea happens after eating, it is due to spleen vacuity. If the feces is loose with totally undigested food, and happens before dawn, it is due to spleen and kidney yang vacuity.

Therapeutic Principle

To supplement the spleen and eliminate dampness is the main therapy for diarrhea. In addition, also treat the causes of diarrhea, such as promoting digestion, resolving accumulation, expelling wind, relieving the exterior, clearing heat, eliminating dampness, strengthening the spleen, supplementing qi and warming the kidney. First treat the complicated patterns of diarrhea when a patient has severe diarrhea.

Differentiation of Patterns

Common Patterns

Food-milk stagnation

Manifestations

Vomiting with undigested food or milk that has a sour odor, abdominal pain that feels better after diarrhea, refusal to eat, fullness and pain of the abdomen, red tongue with yellow and greasy coating, slippery and wiry pulse, or purple and stagnated index vein

Treatment Principle Digest the food and guide down stagnated food, transform the spleen and stop diarrhea.

Formula

Bao He Wan (Harmony Preserving Pills)
    In the formula, Shen Qu(Medicated Leaven), Shan Zha (Frutus Crataegi) and Lai Fu Zi (Semen Raphani Sativi) are for digesting stagnated food and resolving fullness of the abdomen, guiding the stagnated qi and food downwards. Ban Xia (Rhizoma Pinelliae Terntae) and Chen Pi (Pericarpium Citri Reticulatae) harmonize the stomach and eliminate dampness. Lian Qiao (Fructus Forsythiae Suspensae) clears stagnant heat. If the patient has abdominal pain, add Mu Xiang (Radix Aucklandiae Lappae) and Zhi Ke (Bitter Orange Peel).

Exterior evils invading stomach

Manifestations

Loose stool with foam, no severe odor, abdominal pain with borbrygmus, runny nose, aversion to chills and fever, white and greasy coating, floating pulse, reddish index vein.

Treatment Principle Expel wind, release exterior, eliminate dampness and stop diarrhea.

Formula

Huo Xiang Zheng Qi San (Agastache Powder Rectify qi)
    In the formula, Huo Xiang (Agastache) eliminates dampness, regulates qi and harmonizes the middle. Zi Su Ye (Perilla Leaf) and Bai Zhi (Dahurian Angelica Root) expels exterior wind cold and regulates dampness. Ban Xia Rhizoma Pinelliae Ternae) and Chen Pi (Pericarpium Citri Reticulatae) regulate qi and resolve phlegm. Bai Zhu Rhizoma Atractylodis Macrocephalae), Fu Ling (Sclerotium Poriae Cocos) and Zhi Gan Cao (Roasted Licorice) harmonize the middle and resolve dampness. If there is food

stagnation, add Shen Qu (Medicated Leaven) and Shan Zha (Frutus Crataegi) to aid digestion and resolve stagnation.

Diarrhea due to damp-heat

Manifestations

Watery diarrhea with yellow stool, or with mucus, strong odor, abdominal pain, poor appetite, thirst, anxiety, fever, scanty urine, red tongue with yellow and greasy coating, purple index vein.

Treatment Principle Clear heat, eliminate dampness and stop diarrhea

Formula

Ge Gen Qin Lian Tang (Kudzu, Coptis, and Scutellaria Decoction) Ge Ge Radix Puerariae) lifts clear Qi, eliminates dampness, generates body fluid to stop thirst. Huang Qin (Scutellaria Root) and Huang Lian (Rhizoma Coptidis) clear heat, dry dampness and stop diarrhea. Gan Cao(Radix Glycyrrhizae Uralensis) harmonizes the middle. If the heat is worse than the dampness, add Lian Qiao (Fructus Forsythiae Suspensae) and Bai Tou Weng (Pulsatillae Root) to clear heat and toxin. If the dampness is more prevalent than the heat, add Yi Yi Ren (Coix Lachryma-jobi), Bai Bian Dou (Dolichos Lablab), Fu Ling (Sclerotium Poria Cocos) and Che Qian Zi (Plantago Asiatica) to eliminate dampness and stop diarrhea. If there is abdominal fullness, add Hou Po (Cortex Magnoliae Officinalis) and Mu Xiang (Radix Aucklandiae Lappae) to regulate Qi and relieve fullness. If there is vomiting, add Huo Xiang (Agastache) to eliminate dampness and stop vomiting.

Diarrhea due to spleen vacuity

Manifestations

Diarrhea several hours after eating, the feces are clear, loose with undigested food, no bad odor, pale face, tired and weak, weight loss, pale tongue with white coating, thready and weak pulse.

Treatment Principle Strengthen spleen and supplement qi, activate spleen and stop diarrhea.

Formula

Shen Ling Bai Zhu San (Ginseng, Poria, and Atractylodes Macrocephala Powder)

In the formula, Dang Shen (Radix Codonopsitis Pilosulae), Gan Cao (Radix Glycyrrhizae), Fu Ling (Sclerotium Poria Cocos) and Bai Zhu (Rhizoma Atractylodis) strengthen the spleen, nourish the stomach, and supplement the middle Qi. Shan Yao (Radix Dioscoreae Oppositae), Bai Bian Dou (Dolichos Lablab), Lian Zi (Semen Nelumbinis Nuciferae) strengthen the spleen, regulate Qi and harmonize the stomach. Yi Yi Ren (Coix Lachryma-jobi) eliminates dampness and stops diarrhea. Sha Ren (Radix Adenphorae Seu Gleniae) promotes the movement of Qi. If dampness is severe, add Huo Xiang (Agastache) and Pei Lan (Herba Eupatorii Fortunei) to transform dampness. If there is poor appetite, add Mai Ya (Fructus Hordei Vulgaris Germinantus) and Shen Qu (Massa Fermentata) to help digestion. If there is abdominal fullness, add Hou Po (Cortex Magnoliae Officinalis) and Mu Xiang (Radix Aucklandiae Lappae) to regulate Qi and relieve fullness.

Diarrhea due the vacuity of spleen and kidney

Manifestations

Chronic watery diarrhea with undigested food, with prolapsed anus, cold extremities, pale face, tired and weak, pale tongue with white coating, deep and weak pulse.

TreatmentPrinciple Strengthen spleen and supplement qi, strengthen spleen and stop diarrhea.

Formula

Fu Zi Li Zhong Tang (Prepared Aconite Pill to Regulate the Middle) and Si Shen Wan (Four-Miracle pill)

In the formula, Ren Shen (Radix Ginseng), Bai Zhu (Rhizoma Atractylodis) strengthen the spleen and the middle Qi. Gan Jiang (Rhizoma Zinggiberis Officinalis), Wu Zhu Yu (Fructus Evodia Rutaecapae) warm the middle and expel cold. Fu Zi (Radix Aconiti Carmichaeli), Bu Gu Zhi (Fructus Psoraleae), Rou Dou Kou (Fructus Eveodiae Rutaecarpae) and Wu Wei Zi (Fructus Schisandrae Chinensis) warm the kidneys and spleen, bind up the intestine and stop diarrhea. If the patient has prolapsed anus, add Huang Qi (Radix Astragali Membrancei) and Sheng Ma (Rhizoma Cimicifugae) to lift the middle Qi. If there is chronic and severe diarrhea, add He Zi (Fructus Terminaliae Chebulae) to bind up intestine and stop diarrhea.

Complicated Patterns

Dual vacuity of qi and yin

Manifestations

Severe diarrhea, tired and weakness, spiritual malaise, orbital and fontanel depression, or even sunken abdomen, weight loss, anxiety, dry and parched skin, short, scanty urination, red lips, a scarlet red tongue with no fluids, rapid pulse

Treatment principle Supplement qi, nourish yn, and stops diarrhea

Formula

Ren Shen Wu Mei Wan (Ginseng and Mume Pills)

In the formula, *Ren Shen* (Radix Ginseng), *Wu Mei* (Fructus Mume) and *Gan Cao* (Radix Glycyrrhizae) generate Yin. Lian Zi (Semen Nelumbinis Nuciferae) and Shan Yao(Radix Dioscoreae Oppositae) strengthen the spleen and stop diarrhea. If there is chronic diarrhea, add He Zi (Fructus Terminaliae Chebulae) to bind up the intestine and stop diarrhea. If there is thirst and the patient likes to drink water, add Tian Hua Fen (Radix Trichosanthis), Shi Hu (Dendrobium Stem) and Yu Zhu (Rhizoma Polygonti Odorati) to clear heat and generate fluids.

Exhaustion of yin and collapse of yang

Manifestations

Severe diarrhea that is watery and can't be stopped, fatigue, weakness, pale complexion and lack of facial expression, cold extremities, profuse sweating, shortness of breath and sallow breath, pale tongue and faint pulse.

Treatment principle Restore the yang and build up the collapse.

Formula

Shen Fu Long Mu Jiu Ni Tang (Ginseng, Aconite De, Dragon Bone and Oyster Shell Decoction)

In the formula, Ren Shen (Radix Ginseng) strongly supplements Yuan Qi. Zhi Fu Zi (Prepared Radix Aconiti Carmichaeli) restores Yang, Long Gu (Os Draconis) and Mu Li (Concha Ostreae) calms Yang and binds up collapse. Gan Jiang (Rhizoma Zingiberis), Bai Zhu(Rhizoma Atractylodis Macrocephalae) and Zhi Gan Cao (Roasted Licorice) warm the middle, strengthen the spleen and generate Qi.

Other Treatment

Patent herbs

- Huo Xiang Zheng Qi Ye (Agastache Liquid Rectify Qi), taken orally 5ml-10ml for per time, 3 times per day. It is used for diarrhea due to wind cold or damp cold.
- Fu Zi Li Zhong Wan(Prepared Aconite Pill to Regulate the Middle) 0.3g taken orally, 3 times a day. It is used for diarrhea due to vacuity cold of the spleen and Yang.

Acupuncture therapy

Main points: Ren12, St36, UB21, St25. Second points: LI11, St44, Ren6. If there is vomiting, add Ren13, PC6. Reducing technique is for repletion, supplementing technique is for vacuity. Once a day.

Moxibustion Moxa St36, Ren12, Ren8, 7 to 10 for each point, once a day. It is used for diarrhea due to spleen vacuity and Yang vacuity of spleen and kidney.

Tuina

- Diarrhea due to food stagnation kneading Wa Lao Gong and St36, clearing large intestine and Banmen, softening abdomen. 5 to 15 minutes for each point, once every day.
- Diarrhea due to wind cold kneading Wa Lao Gong, pushing San Guan, softening abdomen and umbilicus. 5 to 15 minutes for each point, once every day.
- Diarrhea due to damp heat Pushing Tian He Shui and San Guan, Kneading Xiao Tian Xin and Nei Lao Gong, clearing the large intestine. 5 to 15 minutes for each point, once every day.
- Diarrhea due to spleen vacuity supplementing spleen meridian and large intestine, kneading St36, softening abdomen, pushing Qi Jie Gu. 5 to 15 minutes for each point, once every day.

Topical therapy

Ding Gui San (Clove and Cinnamon Powder). Grind Ding Xiang (Flos Caryophylli)1g and Rou Gui (Cortex Cinnamomi Cassiae)2g as powder, topical use on the umbilicus and cover it with gauze. Once a day. It is used for diarrhea due to cold or vacuity.

Prevention and Care

- Avoid feeding too soon, if the child also has severe vomiting. Gradually feed the food that is easily digested and give a small amount.
- According to climate change, add or reduce the patient's clothes to prevent catching cold.

- keep the bedroom clean and quiet.
- Strongly encourage breastfeeding, carefully and reasonably add General foods.

Constipation (Bian Mi 便秘)

Constipation refers to patients who have a dry stool, prolonged duration between defecation, or dyschezia with no dry stool. It is encountered frequently in the clinic, and occurs all year round. Some of the children may also present with poor appetite and sleep, or even anal fissure or hemorrhoids. Children's constipation is often due to dry heat accumulation or vacuity of Qi and blood, which fails to descend the feces. The main therapy is to nourish intestine and purge the feces. According to the causes of constipation, respectively, dissolve food stagnation, purge the Fu organ, nourish Yin, moisten dryness, supplement Qi and blood. Try to avoid strong herbs, such as Da Huang (Radix et Rhizoma Rhei) and Mang Xiao (Mirabilitum). The formulas, such as Zhi Shi Dao Zhi Wan (Immature Bitter Organge Pill to Guide Out Stagnation), Run Chang Wan (Nourish Intestine Pill) and Ma Zi Ren Wan (Hem Seed Pill) are effective. Tuina, such as purging large intestine and softening abdomen is effective.

Abdominal Pain (Fu Tong 腹 痛)

Abdominal pain is a painful symptom between the stomach and symphysis pubis. Abdominal pain was recorded first in the Huang Di Nei Jing (Yellow Emperor Classic of TCM·), but the children's abdominal pain was first recorded by Chao Yuan Fang in his book, *Zhu Bing Yuan Hou Lun* (General Treatise on the Causes and symptoms of diseases) 610 stated "Children's abdominal pain is often due to disharmony of heat and cold, which cause the heat and cold disturb the Zang and Fu organs. If a patient has reddish complexion, fever, restless, hot hands and feet, it is due to heat. If the patient has pale or purple complexion and lips, it is due to cold. Abdominal pain occurs in a variety of diseases of internal medicine and surgical diseases, occurs at any ages. Infant abdominal pain easy to be misdiagnosed because of some of children can not express correctly. Therefore, a comprehensive and detailed physical examination and laboratory examinations are necessary to confirm the diagnosis.

Etiology and Pathology

- The main causes of abdominal pain are improper diet, exterior pathogenic factors, vacuity of Zang Fu, qi and blood stasis, and round worm blocking the intestines.
- *Invasion of cold pathogen* The cold invades the skin due to improper clothing and stays in the stomach and intestine, or spleen yang is damaged due to having too much cold food. Cold is a yin pathogen, and it constructs muscles, qi and blood, when qi and blood stagnate, there is abdominal pain.
- *Food Stagnation* Children are unable to control their eating on their own. If there is incorrect feeding, or overeating, or having food that is difficult to digest, this injures the spleen and stomach. It fails to transform, and inhibits the ascending and descending of the spleen and stomach, therefore, it causes pain.
- *Vacuity cold of the Zang Fu organs* Damp and cold stay in the interior because of congenital yang vacuity or weak constitution after chronic disease, resulting in qi and blood stagnation, and then pain occurs.
- *Qi and blood stasis* The qi and blood stagnate in the meridians due to trauma, a wound after operation, or chronic diseases, which results in pain.

In summary, abdominal pain may be caused by invasion of cold pathogens, food stagnation, vacuity cold of zang fu organs and qi and blood stasis. The main pathogen is qi and blood stasis. Since abdominal pain can be mixed with repletion and vacuity, it may become critical if incorrectly treated or not treated in a timely manner.

Diagnosis

Diagnostic Guidelines

- The pain occurs in the area that is under stomach, around the umbilicus and above the pubic symphisis.
- It may be acute or chronic.

Differentiation of Diagnosis

- Stomachache It occurs near the center of stomach, it is often accompanied with nausea, vomiting, and acid regurgitation.
- Hypochondriac pain It occurs in the hypochondriac area, there is also distention in the area.

Diagnostic Notes

- Inquiry should focus on age, feeding habits, and understand the triggers of symptoms in detail.
- Try to find the exact location, nature, severity and characteristics of the pain.
- Note whether the abdominal pain is accompanied by fever, jaundice, hematuria, vomiting, diarrhea, blood in the stool.
- During the physical examination, physicians have to palpate the abdomen carefully and comprehensively and as soon as possible rule out whether or not there is a critical disorder. Pay attention if there are abdominal masses, intestinal muscle tension, tenderness, rebound tenderness, and bloating.
- According to the patient's condition, you may do lab exams, such as blood, urine, X-ray, B ultrasound of the abdomen and occult blood of stool.

Pattern Differentiation

Guide lines of differentiation

Differentiating according to the location of abdominal pain

The location of abdominal pain is related to the mechanism of the disease. If the pain is around the navel, it is usually due to round worm. If the pain is all over the abdomen and is dull, it is due to vacuity cold. If there is moving pain, it is due to Qi stagnation. If there is lower right abdominal pain, it is due to the disorder of the large intestine. If the pain is between navel and stomach, it is due to food stagnation.

Differentiating between the causes of abdominal pain

If the pain is acute and is relieved by warming, it is due to cold. If there is fullness and distention that is worse with pressure, it is due to food stagnation. If the pain is chronic and dull, it is due to vacuity cold of the Zang Fu organs. If it is stabbing and distending pain, it is due to stagnation of Qi and blood stasis.

Therapeutic Principle

Regulating qi and unblocking the meridians is the main therapy for abdominal pain. In addition, also treat the causes of it, such as warming the meridian and expelling cold, promoting digestion and resolving accumulation, tonifying the deficiency and removing blood stasis.

Patterns and Treatment

Cold attacking the abdomen

Manifestations

Abdominal pain that is acute, and it is relieved by warming, pale complexion, cold sweating, purple lips when the pain is severe, vomiting and diarrhea, white and greasy tongue coating.

Treatment Principle Warm the cold, expel cold, regulate qi and stop pain.

Formula

Yang Zang Tang (Nourish the Zang Decoction)
    In the formula, Mu Xiang (Radix Aucklandiae Lappae), Ding Xiang (Clove) and Chen Xiang (Aloewood) expel cold and regulate Qi. Dang Gui (Radix Angelicae Sinensis), Chuan Xiong (Radix Lgustici Chuanxiong) warms the meridians and removes blood stasis. If there is nausea and vomiting, add Huo Xiang (Agastache) and Zhu Ru (Phyllostachys Nigra) to harmonize the stomach and stop vomiting. If there is severe abdominal pain, also add Yan Hu Suo (Corydalis Yanhusuo) to regulate Qi and stop pain.

Food-milk stagnation

Manifestations

Abdominal fullness that is worse with pressure, vomiting with undigested food or milk that has a sour odor, and loose stool that has a rotten odor, poor appetite, gas, restless sleep, thick and greasy tongue coating, slippery and rapid pulse, purple and stagnated index vein.

Treatment Principle Digest the food and guide stagnated food downwards, transform the spleen and stop pain.

Formula

Bao He Wan (Harmony Preserving Pills)
    In the formula, Shen Qu (Medicated Leaven), Shan Zha (Frutus Crataegi) and Lai Fu Zi (Semen Raphani Sativi) digest stagnated food and resolve abdominal fullness. Zhi ke (Bitter Orange Peel), Chen Pi (Pericarpium Citri Reticulatae) regulate qi and stop pain. If there is constipation, add Bing Lang (Semen Arecae Catechu).

Vacuity cold of the Zang and Fu

Manifestations

Dull pain that is sometimes worse and sometime better, it is better when it is pressed and warmed, it is also better after eating, pale complexion, poor appetite, loose stool, cold extremities, pale tongue with thin white coating, pale and deep index vein.

Treatment Principle Warm the middle and supplement the vacuity, regulate qi and stop pain.

Formula

Xiao Jian Zhong Tang (Minor Construct the Middle Decoction) and Li Zhong Tang (Regulate the Middle Decoction)

In the formula, Gui Zhi (Ramulus Cinnamomi Cassiae) warms the meridians and harmonies the Ying, Bai Shao (Radix Paeoniae Lactiflorae) and Gan Cao (Radix Glycyrrhizae Uralensis) rela tendons and stop pain, Sheng Jiang (Rhizoma Zingiberis Officinalis Recens), Da Zao (Fructus Zizphi Jujubae), Dang Shen (Radix Codonopsitis Pilosulae) and Bai Zhu (Rhizoma Atractylodis) supplement the middle, Gan Jiang (Dried Rhizoma Zinggiberis Officinalis) warms the middle and expels cold. If there is qi and blood vacuity, add Huang Qin (Radix Scutellariae Baicalensis) and Dang Gui (Radix Angelicae Sinensis). If there is kidney Yang vacuity, add Fu Zi (Radix Aconiti Carmichaeli) and Rou Gui (Cortex Cinnamomi Cassiae). If there is severe cold pain in the abdomen, add Wu Zhu Yu (Fructus Evodia Rutaecapae)

Qi and blood stasis

Manifestations

Stabbing abdominal pain that is worse with pressure, or abdominal mass that is not moveable, purple lips and tongue,

Treatment Principle Remove blood stasis, regulate qi and stop pain.

Formula

Shao Fu Zhu Yu Tang (Drive out Blood Stasis from Lower Abdomen)
In the formula, Rou Gui (Cortex Cinnamomi Cassiae), Gan
Jiang (Dried Rhizoma Zinggiberis Officinalis) and Xiao Hui Xiang
(Common Fennel Fruit) warms the meridians and opens the
channels, Wu Ling Zhi (Excrementum Trogopteri Seu Pteromi),
Pu Huang (Pollen Typhae) and Chi Shao (Radix Paeoniae Rubra),
Dang Gui (Radix Angelicae Sinensis) and Chuang Xiong (Radix
Ligustici Chuanxiong) remove blood stasis, Yan Hu Suo (Corydalis
Yanhusuo) and Mo Yao (Myrrha) regulate qi and remove blood
stasis. If there is distention and pain, add Wu Yao (Lindera Root)
and Chuan Lian Zi (Melia Toosendan). If there is a mass, add San
Leng (Rhizoma Sparganii)

Other Treatment

Patent herbs

- Huo Xiang Zheng Qi Ye (Agastache Liquid Rectify Qi),
  taken orally 5ml~10ml for per time, 3 times per day. It is
  used for abdominal pain due to cold attacking abdomen.
- Fu Zi Li Zhong Wan(Prepared Aconite Pill to Regulate
  the Middle) 0.3g taken orally, 3 times a day. It is used for
  abdominal pain due to vacuity cold of Zang Fu.

Acupuncture

Points: Ren12, St36, LI4. If there is cold in the abdomen, also add
moxa at Ren8. If there is food stagnation, also add St44. If there
is vomiting, add PC6. Once a day.

Tuina

If the abdominal pain is due to cold, perform kneading at Wai Lao
Gong and Yi Wo Feng. If it is due to food stagnation, clear the
spleen and stomach, transform Ba Gua, clear large intestine and
Ban Men. 5 to 15 minutes for each point, once every day.

Topical therapy

Ding Gui San (Clove and Cinnamon Powder). Grind Ding Xiang (Flos Caryophylli) 1g and Rou Gui(Cortex Cinnamomi Cassiae) 2g into a powder, use topically on the umbilicus, cover it with gauze. Once a day, it is used for abdominal pain due to cold or vacuity.

Prevention and care

Avoid eating cold foods and drinking cold water. Pay attention to keep the abdomen warm.

Lack of Appetite (Yan Shi 厌食)

Lack of appetite is a syndrome referring to the child who has no desire to eat, no appetite, or even refuses to eat. This syndrome occurs in all ages of childhood, but it has a higher incident between 1~6 years old, especially the children who live in cities. It doesn't have an obvious seasonal component. Most children only lose appetite, no other symptoms. However, if the problem persists, there may be weight loss or malnutrition. There is not much information in ancient texts devoted to this syndrome, a few of them discussed the syndrome as "dislike food", "no desire to eat".

Etiology and Pathology

The main causes of lack of appetite are improper diet and incorrect nursing after diseases which affect the stomach's function of receiving food and the spleen's function of transformation.

Improper diet

Parents who are lacking scientific nursing knowledge may lead to children being fed foods that are too greasy and sweet or addicted to food, or excessive feeding. All of these will injure the spleen and stomach, affecting the stomach's receiving function, leading to a lack of appetite.

Incorrect nursing after diseases

After suffering diseases, such as febrile diseases, the child has qi and yin vacuity of the spleen and stomach, which affects the spleen and stomach function, resulting in failure of the stomach receiving food, and the lack of appetite occurs.

Diagnosis

Diagnostic guidelines

- Chronic lack of appetite with no other diseases.
- The child has pale complexion, be slightly slim, but the spirit and health are still good
- The child has an improper feeding history, such as eating irregularly, too much or too little quantity, excessive eating cold, sweet and greasy food and snacks.

Pattern Differentiation

Guidelines of differentiation

Differentiating the patterns is important for this syndrome. If there is only poor appetite and no other symptoms, it is due to disharmony between the stomach and spleen. If there is also a pale complexion and loose stool, it is due to qi vacuity of the stomach and spleen. If there is also a red tongue with a peeled coating and thirst, preference for cold water, it is due to yin vacuity of the stomach and spleen.

Therapeutic Principle

To increase appetite and transform the spleen is the main therapy for lack of appetite. You may add harmonizing the stomach and transforming spleen, supplementing the spleen qi and nourishing the stomach yin according to the pattern differentiation.

Patterns and Treatment

Disharmony between the stomach and spleen

Manifestations

Lack of appetite, even refusing to eat, the child will have fullness and distention of the abdomen if he is forced to eat, slightly slim, slight pale complexion, good spirit, pale tongue with thin and white or white and greasy coating, pale index vein and slippery pulse.

Treatment Principle Harmonize the stomach and transform spleen.

Formula

Tiao Pi San (Regulate the Spleen Powder)
    In the formula, Cang Zhu (Rhizoma Atractylodis) transforms the spleen and dries dampness, Chen Pi (Pericarpium Citri Reticulatae) regulates qi and dries dampness, Ji Nei Jin (Endithelium Corneum) and Shen Qu (Massa Fermentata) help digest the food and increase appetite, Pei lan (Herba Eupatorii) eliminates dampness and transforms thee is abdominal fullness, add Yi Yi Ren(Coix Lachryma-jobi) and Huo Xiang (Agastache) to eliminate dampness and strengthen the spleen.

Qi vacuity of the stomach and spleen

Manifestations

Poor appetite, tired and weak, pale complexion, loose stool with undigested food, pale tongue with thin and white coating, weak pulse.

Treatment Principle Transform the spleen and supplement qi

Formula

Shen Ling Bai Zhu San(Ginseng, Poria, and Atractylodes Macrocephala Powder)

In the formula, the four gentlemen is used for supplementing qi. Shan Yao (Radix Dioscoreae Oppositae), Bai Bian Dou (Dolichos Lablab), Lian Zi (Semen Nelumbinis Nuciferae) strengthen the spleen, regulate qi and harmonize the stomach. Yi Yi Ren (Coix Lachryma-jobi) and Sha Ren (Radix Adenphorae Seu Gleniae) eliminate dampness and promote the movement of Qi. If there is loose stool, add He Zi (Fructus Terminaliae Chebulae) Wu Mei (Fructus Mume) to bind up the intestine and stop diarrhea. If there is weak energy and susceptibility to illness, also add Huang Qi (Radix Astragali Membranaceus) and Mu Li (Concha Ostreae) to strengthen Wei Qi.

Yin vacuity of the spleen and stomach

Manifestations

Poor appetite, dry mouth and thirst, desire to drink cold water, pale and dull complexion, constipation, yellow urine, red tongue with less coating or peeled coating, thin and rapid pulse.

Treatment Principle Nourish the stomach yin

Formula

Yang Wei Zen Ye Tang (Nourish the Stomach and Generate Yin Decoction)

In the formula, Sha Shen (Radix Denophorae Strictae), Mai Men Dong (Tuber Ophiopogonis Japonici) and Shi Hu (Dendrobium Stem) clear the lung and generate the stomach, Yu Zhu (Rhizoma Polygonti Odorati) and Bai Shao (Radix Paeoniae Lactiflorae) clear heat, generate fluids and supplement blood. It there are red and dry lips, add Tian Hua Fen (Radix Trichosanthis) and Lu Gen (Rhizoma Phragmitis Communis). If there are hot palms and night sweating, add Mu Dan Pi (Cortex Moutan Radicis) and Di Gu Pi (Cortex Lycii Radicis). If there is constipation, add Da Huang (Radix et Rhizoma Rhei) and Huo Ma Ren (Semen Cannabis Sativae).

Other Treatment

Patent herbs

- Qu Mai Zhi Zhu Wan (Medicated Leaven, Barley Sprout, Immature Bitter Orange, and Atractylodes Macrocephala Pill), taken orally 1 pill for per time, 3 times per day. It is used for the syndrome of disharmony.
- Xia Er Jian Pi Wan(Pediatric Transforming Spleen Pills) 1 pill taken orally, 3 times a day. It is used for the syndrome of spleen and stomach vacuity.

Tuina

- Push and tonify the spleen for 2 minutes, knead Yi Wo Feng for 3 minutes, divide Yin and Yang 2 minutes, transform Nei Ba Gua for 4 minutes, clear Tian He Shui 1 minutes.
- Once a day, 14 days is one cause of treatment. It is used for disharmony of the spleen and stomach.

Topical therapy

Gao Liang Jiang (Galangal), Qing Pi (Pericarpium Citri Reticulatae Viride), Chen Pi (Pericarpium Citri Reticulatae), Cang Zhu (Rhizoma Atractylodis), Bo He (Herba Menthae Haplocalycis) and Chuan Jiao (Pericarpium Zanthoxyly Bungeani). Each of them is same dosage, make them as powder and put it into bag. Place it on the abdomen.

Prevention and care

- Feed and educate the children properly, feed them more vegetables, and offer a variety of foods.

- Avoid drinking too much water just before or during feeding.
- Try to create a good eating environment, void crying before feeding.

The Syndrome of Indigestion (Ji Zhi 积滞)

Indigestion is a syndrome of the spleen and stomach. It is due to improper feeding of milk or food that can't be digested and the food accumulates with qi stagnation in the middle Jiao. It is manifested by no appetite, fullness and distention of the abdomen, acid reflux, or vomiting and diarrhea with indigestion. The syndrome was first recorded in *Yin Tong Bai Wen* (One Hundred Questions about Childhood) states "If a child has the syndrome of indigestion, he may have a pale and puffy complexion, painful and hot abdomen, tired, crying, poor appetite, constipation, greasy urine, loose stool that is white with a strong sour smell. " It may happen at any age, but the incidence is higher under 3 years of age. The syndrome of indigestion has a close relationship with malnutrition. *You You Ji Chen* (A Collection of Pediatrics) by Chen Fu Zhen in 1750 states "A child has food stagnation; it may cause the syndrome of indigestion if the food stagnation hasn't been cured in time. The syndrome of indigestion may also result in malnutrition if the indigestion hasn't been cured in time. " If the food injuring the body hasn't been cured, it will develop into indigestion syndrome. If the indigestion still hasn't been cured, it will result in malnutrition manifested by emaciation and slow development.

Etiology and Pathology

Food stagnation or vacuity of the spleen and stomach is the main cause of indigestion.

Food Stagnation A child is not robust and the stomach is small and tender and cannot contain large amounts of food. If patients are nursed and fed even slightly inappropriately, this will result in food retention and qi stagnation in the middle Jiao.

Vacuity of Spleen and stomach Incorrect feeding or nursing of a child after suffering diseases, results in the failure to digest food. There may also be underlying vacuity of the spleen and stomach.

In summary, the syndrome of indigestion is due to food and milk stagnation, or vacuity of the spleen and stomach, which results in food and qi stagnation in the middle Jiao.

Diagnosis

Diagnostic Guidelines

There is a history of improper feeding. The child has no appetite, fullness and distention of the abdomen, acid reflux, or vomiting and diarrhea with undigested food. It may be accompanied by anxiety and irritability, crying during the night, milky urine.

Differentiation of Diagnosis

- Lack of appetite A child only has lack of appetite in long term, but still has good spirit, and no other diseases.
- Malnutrition A child is obviously slim, accompanied with other symptoms of spleen, stomach, spirit and nervous system.

Diagnostic Notes

- Gain understanding of the child's age, nursing ways, and diet.
- Know if there is a history of vomiting, diarrhea. Pay attention of location and nature of the abdominal pain.
- Carefully check the spirit, complexion, lips tongue and tongue coating of the patient. Palpate the abdomen of the child.

Pattern Differentiation

Guidelines of differentiation

Focus on differentiating between the repletion and vacuity pattern of indigestion. If there is abdominal fullness and pain that dislikes pressure, vomiting immediately after eating, that is sour and has a bad smell, the patient feels better after defecation, red tongue with thick and greasy coating, it belongs to a repletion pattern. On the other hand, if there is abdominal fullness without pain that likes pressure, the patient has a pale complexion, tired and loose stools, pale tongue with thin white coating, is is vacuity pattern.

Therapeutic Principle

The basic therapy is to reduce food stagnation. If it is a repletion pattern, add the herbs that clear heat and purge the Fu organs. If it is a vacuity pattern, add the herbs that supplement the spleen and stomach.

Patterns and treatment

Food stagnation

Manifestation

Abdominal fullness, acid regurgitation, poor appetite, sour stool, crying, anxiety, cloudy urine, red tongue with greasy coating, slippery and wiry pulse

Treatment Principle

Reduce food stagnation and harmonize stomach

Formula

Bao He Wan (Preserve harmony Pill)

In the formula, Shen Qu (Medicated Leaven), Shan Zha (Frutus Crataegi) and Lai Fu Zi (Semen Raphani Sativi) digest stagnated food and resolve fullness of the abdomen, guiding the stagnated qi and food downwards. Ban Xia (Rhizoma Pinelliae Terntae) and Chen Pi (Pericarpium Citri Reticulatae) harmonizes the stomach and eliminates dampness. Lian Qiao (Fructus Forsythiae Suspensae) clears heat. If the patient has abdominal pain, add Mu Xiang (Radix Aucklandiae Lappae) and Zhi Ke (Bitter Orange Peel).

Vacuity of the spleen and stomach

Manifestations

Pale complexion, slim body, fatigue, restlessness, poor appetite, loose stool, pale tongue with white and greasy coating, pale index vein, thin and slippery pulse.

Treatment Principle Strengthen the spleen and reduce food stagnation

Formula

Xiao Er Jian Pi Wan (Pediatric Transforming Spleen Pills)
    In the formula, Dang Shen (Radix Ccodonopsitis Pilosulae) and Bai Zhu (Rhizoma Atractylodis) strengthen the spleen Qi. Shen Qu (Medicated Leaven), Shan Zha (Frutus Crataegi) and Mai Ya (Fructus Hordei Vulgaris Germinantus) for reduce food stagnation. Chen Pi (Pericarpium Citri Reticulatae) and (Fructus Immaturus Citri Aurantii) regulate Qi and resolve abdominal distention. If there is vomiting, add Ban Xia (Rhizoma Pinelliae Ternae) and Sheng Jiang (Rhizoma Zingiberis Officinalis Recens) to harmonize the stomach. If there is loose stool, add Pao Jiang (Quick-fried Rhizoma Zingiberis Officinalis) and Wu Mei (Fructus Pruni Mume) to warm the middle Jiao and stop diarrhea.

Other Treatment

Patent herbs

- Xia Er Hua Shi Wan(Eeduce the Food Stagnation Pill for Children), taken orally 1 pill for per time, 3 times per day. It is used for food stagnation.
- Bao He Wan(Preserve Harmony Pill) 1 pill taken orally, 3 times a day. It is used for food stagnation.
- Xiao Er Jian Pi Wan(Pediatric Transforming Spleen Pills) 1 pill taken orally, 3 times a day. It is used for spleen vacuity with food stagnation.

Acupuncture

Puncture St36, Ren12, Ren6, UB25, UB20, UB21 for spleen vacuity with food stagnation. Puncture Si Feng for spleen vacuity with food stagnation.

Tuina

- Repletion syndrome Push and knead Banmen, clear large intestine, knead Ren12, Ren8 and St36. 50 times for each of them. Pinch spine 3 times.
- Vacuity syndrome Push and supplement the spleen, transform the water to the earth, knead Ren 12, Wai Lao Gong and St36. Each for 50 times. You may also knead the spine.

Topical therapy

Mix Shen Qu (Medicated Leaven), Mai Ya (Fructus Hordei Vulgaris Germinantus) and Shan Zha (Frutus Crataegi), each of them 30g, Bing Lang (Semen Arecae Catechu) and Da Huang (Radix et Rhizoma Rhei)10g, Mang Xiao (Mirabilitum)20g with sesame oil. Put the herbs at Ren12 and Ren8. Keep it for 24 hours, 1/2days. Three times is one course of treatment. It is used for food stagnation with abdominal pain.

Prevention and care

- Strongly advocate mother to breastfeed their babies, feed child regularly. Add solid in time, feed infant reasonably, and the food should be nutritious and easily digestible.
- One should avoid feeding food that is too greasy, fatty, or sweet food. Try do not give candy and cookies, but feed more vegetables, and train children to eat healthy food.

Malnutrition (Gan Syndrome 疳积)

Malnutrition is a chronic disease that gradually results from improper feeding or from the impact of other diseases, such that it damages the spleen and stomach, and injures the qi and body fluids. It is characterized by emaciation, sallow complexion, abnormal appetite, hair loss, tired and apathetic, or dysphoria. Its onset is without a relationship with the seasons, it is more common in children under 5 years of age. It was listed as one the worst diseases in ancient times. Gan in Chinese has two meanings. "Gan means sweet" the cause of Gan results from improper diet that includes feeding too many greasy, fatty and sweet foods. "Gan means dryness", it refers to the pathology and its manifestations. The main pathology is dryness of the body fluid and consumption of qi and blood. The main manifestations are shriveled body and extreme emaciation.

Gan syndrome was recorded first in the Sui dynasty, *Zhu Bing Yuan Huo Lun* (General Treatise on the Causes and symptoms of disease) by Chao Yuan-fang, 610 states "heat oversteams the body, it will consume the five zang and results in Gan syndrome". Dr. Qian Yi, song dynasty 1119 in his book, *Xiao Er Yue Zheng Zhi Jue* (Key to Differentiation and Treatment of Disease of Children) stated: "Malnourishment mostly belongs to the diseases of the spleen and stomach, resulting from vacuity of body fluid. " He recognized the location of malnutrition as being in the spleen and stomach. The ancient physicians classified malnutrition according to the five zang organs, such as the spleen Gan, liver Gan, heart Gan, lung Gan and kidney Gan. The incidence of malnutrition has been decreased significantly in recent years and the clinical symptoms have abated. In Western medicine, The Gan syndrome includes all nutritional disorders caused by a variety of diseases.

Etiology and Pathology

The main cause of malnutrition is improper feeding or the impact of the other diseases. The main pathology is that the spleen and stomach are damaged, and an interruption of transformation and transportation of the spleen and stomach, which causes the insufficient production of qi, blood and body fluid

Prolonged diseases

A physician, Xia Ding stated in his book, *You Ke Tie Jing* (Iron Mirror for pediatrics, 1695) stated "Malnutrition is caused by insufficient spleen and stomach function and consumption of fluid and qi due to chronic vomiting, cough, diarrhea, dysentery and sores". In addition, the parasites were also a main cause of malnutrition in ancient times.

Because the spleen and stomach fail to produce the qi and blood they become insufficient; this will gradually damage the other organs and lead to complications. For example, it will result in Yan Gan (malnutrition of eyes) if the yang of the liver becomes hyperascendent due to the spleen vacuity. It will cause Kou Gan (mouth ulcer) if the liver fire stirs up along the meridian due to the heart fire flaring up resulting from the spleen disorder affecting the heart. If there is spleen qi vacuity, it fails to control the blood in the vessels, it may cause purple spots. At the end of the disease, the disorder of the spleen will involve the kidney, and damage the Yuan qi of the kidney, which causes exhaustion of yin and yang.

Diagnosis

Diagnostic Guidelines

- There is a history of a child who is fed incorrectly or has chronic diseases that became chronic.
- The child has emaciation, he is lower than the normal value of 15% to 40% of body weight, pale complexion, sparse hair. In severe cases, his body weight is even less than 40% of the normal value. The patient also has the dysfunction of the spleen and stomach, such as abnormal appetite, abnormal bowl movement that present as diarrhea or constipation, and belly expansion. The patient has tiredness, or short temper, irritability, frequent rubbing of the eyes, or sucking fingers and grinding teeth.

Differentiation of Diagnosis

- Lack of appetite A child only has a lack of appetite for a long term, but still has good spirit, and no other diseases.
- Indigestion Syndrome The main manifestations are no appetite, fullness and distention of abdomen, acid reflux, or vomiting and diarrhea with indigestion.

Diagnostic Notes

- First, know the nutrition of the child, such as evaluate the weight and fat of under skin, carefully observe the state of the complexion and spirit, skin hair and nails.
- Know the time and rate of the child's weight loss, whether they have loss of appetite, diarrhea, night sweats and other medical history.
- Carefully ask breeds, delivery and feeding history.
- Blood test is recommended if necessary.

Pattern Differentiation

Guidelines of differentiation

- Differentiation between mild or severe disease
- If it is mild disease, has a short history, the manifestations are mild, such as pale face, poor appetite, thinning hair, short temper. If it is a severe case, with a long history, the manifestations are severe, such as
- Severe emaciation, body mass is lower than the normal value of 15% to 40% of body weight, frequent rubbing of the eyes, or sucking fingers and grinding teeth.

Therapeutic Principle

The basic therapy is to strengthen the spleen and stomach. Common therapies are harmonizing the stomach, transforming spleen, digesting the food stagnation and transforming the spleen, supplementing the qi and blood. Also note treating the complications of malnutrition.

Patterns and Treatment

Gan Qi (Failure of spleen's transportation)

Manifestations

Mild emaciation, pale complexion, poor appetite, thinning hair, short temper, diarrhea or constipation, pale tongue with thin coating, thin pulse.

Treatment Principle Harmonize the stomach and transform the spleen.

Formula

Zi Sheng Jian Pi Wan (Enrich the Spleen Pill)
    In the formula, Dang Shen (Radix Codonopsitis Pilosulae), Fu Ling (Sclerotium Poria Cocos) and Bai Zhu (Rhizoma Atractylodis), Bai Bian Dou (Dolichos Lablab), Lian Zi (Semen Nelumbinis Nuciferae) and Shan Yao (Radix Dioscoreae Oppositae) strengthen the spleen, nourish the stomach, supplement the middle qi. Yi Yi Ren (Coix Lachryma-jobi) eliminates dampness and supplements the spleen. Shen Qu (Massa Fermentata) and Shan Zha (Frutus Crataegi) aid digestion. If there is diarrhea, add Pao Jiang (Quick-fried Rhizoma Zingiberis Officinalis). If there is constipation, add Huo Ma Ren (Semen Cannabis Sativae) and Lai Fu Zi (Semen Raphani Sativi).

Spleen vacuity with stagnation

Manifestations

Obvious emaciation, belly expansion, poor appetite, thinning and dry hair, short temper, restlessness, frequent rubbing of the eyes, sucking fingers, grinding teeth, a lot bowel movement, pale tongue with thick and greasy coating, thin and a rapid pulse.

Treatment Principle Harmonize the spleen and stomach, relieve dyspepsia.

Formula

Fei Er Wan (Enrich the Children Pill).

In the formula, Dang Shen (Radix Codonopsitis Pilosulae), Fu Ling (Sclerotium Poria Cocos) and Bai Zhu (Rhizoma Atractylodis) transform the spleen and eliminate dampness. Hu Huang Lian(Rhizoma Picrorrhizae) clears vacuous heat of the heart. Shi Jun Zi (Fructus Quisqualis Indicae) kills the parasites. Mai Ya (Fructus Hordei Vulgaris Germinantus), Shen Qu (Massa Fermentata) and Gu Ya(Fructus Oryzae Sativae Germinantus) aid digestion. If there is thirst and a desire to drink, add Shi Hu (Dendrobium Stem), Tian Hua Fen (Radix Trichosanthes). If there is abdominal pain, add Mu Xiang (Radix Aucklandiae Lappae) and Zhi Ke (Bitter Orange Peel). If there is a red tongue with a peeled coating, hot palms, add Sheng Di Huang (Radix Rehmanniae Glutinosae) and Mu Dan Pi (Cortex Moutan Radicis).

Qi and blood vacuity

Manifestations

Extremely emaciated, shriveled and dry skin, the patient's complexion looks very old, there is only skin covering the bones but no muscle, very weak and dull eye spirit, no tears when the child cries, abdomen is concave shaped like a boat, no appetite at all, red and dry lips,

Treatment Principle Supplement the qi and blood.

Formula

Ba Zhen Tang (Eight Tressures Decoction)

In the formula, the four gentlemen and four ladies are used harmonize and supplement Qi and blood. If there is Yin vacuity of the stomach, add Wu Mei (Fructus Pruni Mume) and Shi Hu

(Dendrobium Stem). If there is Yang vacuity of the spleen and kidney, add Fu Zi (Radix Aconiti Carmichaeli) and Gan Jiang Rhizoma Zinggiberis Officinalis). If the whole body is exhaustive, Sheng Mai San (Generate Pulse Powder) is recommended. If the patient had a collapse syndrome, Shen Fu Long Mu Jiu Ni Tang (Ginseng, Aconite De, Dragon Bone and Oyster Shell Decoction) should be used immediately.

Complicated Patterns

The severe Gan Ji may have the following complications:

Yan Gan (The malnutrition of eyes)

Manifestations

In addition to the original manifestations of malnutrition, the patient also has photophobia, dry and itching eyes, dull eyes, opacity of aqueous humor, cortical peripheral opacity of the lens, night blindness.

Treatment Principle Strengthen the spleen and generate blood, nourish yin and benefit the eyes.

Formula

Shen Ling Bai Zhu San and Shi Hu Yi Guang Wan (Ginseng, Poria, and Atractylodes Macrocephala Powder and Dendrobium Pill for Night Vision)

In the formula, Shen Ling Bai Zhu San strengthens the spleen and stomach. Shi Hu (Dendrobium Stem), Tian Men Dong (Tuber Asparagi Cochinensis) and Sheng Di Huang (Radix Rehmanniae Glutinosae) nourish Yin and supplement kidney. Ling Yang Jiao (Cornu Antelopis),Qing Xiang Zi (Semen Celosiae Argenteae), Huang Lian (Rhizoma Coptidis) clear the heart fire and brighten the eyes. Rou Cong Rong (Herba Cistanches Deserticolae) and Tu Si Zi (Semen Cuscutae Chinesis) supplement the liver and kidneys. Zhi ke (Bitter Orange Peel) and Chuan Xiong (Radix Lgustici Chuanxiong) regulate Qi and remove blood stasis.

Kou Gan (Malnutrition of Mouth)

Manifestations

In addition to the original manifestations of malnutrition, the patient also has sores in the mouth and tongue, or oral erosions with a foul smell, red face and lips, irritability, crying, feared, anxiety, red tongue, thin yellow coating.

Treatment Principle Strengthen the spleen and generate blood, clear the heart and purge fire.

Formula

Shen Ling Bai Zhu San and Dao Chi San (Ginseng, Poria, and Atractylodes macrocephala Powder and Guide Red Powder)
   In the formula, Shen Ling Bai Zhu San strengthens the spleen and stomach and Huang Lian (Rhizoma Coptidis), Tong Cao (Tetrapanax Papyriferus) clears heat and fire of the heart, Sheng Di Huang (Radix Rehmanniae Glutinosae) nourishes yin. If there is scanty urine, also add Hua Shi (Talcum) and Dan Zhu Ye (Herba Lophatheri) to promote urination and to clear the heart heat. If there is thirst, add Shi Hu (Dendrobium Stem) and Yu Zhu (Rhizoma Polygonti Odorati) to nourish yin, generate fluids and clear fire.

Gan Zhong Zhang (Edema due to Malnutrition)

Manifestations

In addition to the original manifestations of malnutrition, the patient also has pitting edema, puffy and cold extremities, less urine and loose stool, pale tongue with white coating.

Treatment principle Strengthen the spleen, warm yang and promote urination.

Formula

Shen Ling Bai Zhu San and Zhen Wu Tang(Ginseng, Poria, and Atractylodes macrocephala Powder and True Warrior Decoction)

In the formula, Shen Ling Bai Zhu San strengthens the spleen and stomach, add Fu Zi (Radix Aconiti Carmichaeli) for warming Yang and promoting urination, Sheng Jiang (Rhizoma Zingiberis Officinalis Recens), Bai Shao (Radix Paeoniae Lactiflorae) warm the middle and expel cold.

Other Treatment

Patent herbs

- Fei Er Wan(Fat Baby pill), taken orally 1 pill per time, 3 times per day. It is used for the syndrome of spleen vacuity with hyperactivity of liver and food stagnation with accumulation of parasites.

Acupuncture

Puncture St36, Ren12, Ren6, UB25, UB20, UB21 for spleen vacuity with food stagnation. Puncture Si Feng for spleen vacuity with food stagnation.

Tuina

- Push San Guan (three gates), reduce six Fu, devide yin and yang, transforming the spleen, soften Ban Men, Sp9, St36, Ub21 and abdomen. It is used for Gan Qi. Pinch spine, especially with strong lifting at Du14, Ub20 and Ub21.
- Prick to bleed, or squeeze out a small amount of yellowish fluid locally from Si Feng. Once a day, until there is no more yellowish fluid out from the point.

Topical therapy

- Mix Da Huang (Radix et Rhizoma Rhei), Mang Xiao (Mirabilitum), Zhi Zi (Fructus Gardeniae Jasminoidis), Xing Ren (Semen Pruni Armeniacae) and Tao Ren (Semen Persica), each of them 6g with flour, onion and vinegar. Make a paste and put it on the umbilicus. Once a day, for 3-5 days. It is used for Gan Ji (Spleen vacuity with stagnation).
- Prepare Lai Fu Zi (Semen Raphani Sativi)3g as a granule and mix it with water, then put on the umbilicus. Once a day, for 7 days. It is used for Gan Ji (Spleen vacuity with stagnation).

Prevention and care

- Strongly advocate mothers to breastfeed their babies, feed in quantitative and timely.
- Prevent children from becoming addicted to a particular food or overeating. Add solid foods in time, feed infant reasonably, the food should be nutritious and easily digestible.
- Do physical examinations regularly to observe if the growth in the children is normal. If there is a nutritive issue, visit doctors, so that the child can be early diagnosed and treated

Children Overweight and Obesity
(Xiao Er Fei Pang Zheng 小儿肥胖症)

Overweight and obesity are the result of "caloric imbalance", too few calories expended for the amount of calories consumed. Overweight is excess body weight for a particular height from fat, muscle, bone, water, or a combination of these factors. Obesity is defined as having excess body fat. The percentage of children aged 6–11 years in the United States who were obese increased from 7% in 1980 to nearly 18% in 2010. Similarly, the percentage of adolescents aged 12~19 years who were obese increased from 5% to 18% over the same period (NIH, 2011, 2012). With the development of overweight and obesity, the children are at risk for a number of conditions, including high cholesterol, high blood pressure, early heart disease, diabetes, sleep apnea, bone problems, skin conditions, heat rash, fungal infections, and acne.

Etiology and Pathology

- Spleen vacuity with damp-phlegm
- Young children's spleen and stomach are generally considered insufficient. If, in addition, the child suffers from a chronic disease such as diarrhea or vomiting, the spleen will fail in its function of transformation and transportation of food. The food will then transform into dampness and phlegm, resulting in obesity.
- Excessive intake fats and sweets
- Pregnant woman have damp phlegm accumulation in body due to addiction to sweet or greasy foods during pregnancy, which results in damp phlegm accumulating in the fetus. Or the child has been fed by too much greasy and sweet food, which leads to damp and phlegm stagnation in the body and obesity occurs.

Pattern Differentiation

Spleen vacuity with damp-phlegm

Manifestations

Overweight, lassitude, heaviness, abdominal fullness, edema, pale complexion, loose feces, swollen and pale tongue with thin coating, deep and slippery pulse.

Treatment Principle Strengthen the spleen, eliminate dampness and resolve phlegm

Formula

Ling Gui Zhu Gan Tang (Poria, Cinnamon Twig, Atractylodes Macrocephala, and Licorice Decoction)

Acupuncture

St36, Qi Si Bian, St40, Sp9. Tuina: soft abdomen, push spleen

Damp-heat of the spleen and stomach

Manifestations

Overweight, head distention, vertigo, overeating, foul breath, constipation, red lips and tongue with yellow greasy coating, slippery and rapid pulse.

Treatment Principle Strengthen the spleen, eliminate dampness and resolve phlegm

Formula

Xie Huang San (Purge Yellow Powder) or Da Chen Qi Tang (Major Order Qi Decoction)

Acupuncture

St44, LI 11, Sp4, St 25, Qi Si Bian. Sweet point. Tuina: Pruge stomach and Tian He Shui.

Diseases and Syndromes of the Heart and Liver

The diseases and syndromes of the heart and liver are mainly located in the heart and liver. The heart is considered to be the emperor, it houses the mind, dominates the blood and vessels; which means it provides the motive force for blood circulation,. It is also in charge of cognition and spirit. The liver stores the soul (Hun) and blood, it maintains the free flow of qi, it is responsible for comfortable, free-going and harmonious functional activity of qi, emotion, blood and the zang fu organs. Therefore, the heart and liver coordinate to regulate the movement of spirit, emotion, qi and blood. The heart and liver are commonly in surplus during childhood. The heart fire is easy to be stirred up, and liver wind tends to stir inside the body. This is why children often have convulsion syndromes when they have fever. The disorders of the heart and liver have increased in recent years. Disorders such as attention deficient disorder (ADD) and attention deficient hyperactivity disorder (ADHD). The main therapy is to calm the liver and heart, invigorate the blood, and quiet the spirit and emotions.

Children's Convulsion
(Xiao Er Jing Feng 小儿惊风)

This is a critical and emergent syndrome manifested with convulsions and with coma. It is more common under 6 years of age. It is one of the four critical syndromes in ancient times. It is a ferocious and critical condition with a high rate of incidence. The

169

symptoms, causes and pathology of convulsion was mentioned in *Huang Di Nei Jing* (Yellow Classic of Chinese Medicine) it states "All the syndromes of trembling and dizziness caused by the wind evil are pertaining to the liver, all the syndromes of convulsive (opisthotonus) disease and stiffness of the neck are pertaining to wetness, and all syndromes of sudden muscular stiffness are pertaining to the wind evil". This disorder was identified as epilepsy as Jing (convulsion) and Xian (epilepsy) before the Song dynasty. It started out as acute and chronic convulsions in the book, *Taiping Benevolent Prescription in North Song dynasty*, AD 992. Qian Yi, a pediatrician, in his book, *Xiao Er Yao Zheng Zhi Yue* (Key to Differentiation and Treatment of Disease of Children) mentioned that the location of acute convulsion is in the heart and liver, but chronic convulsions occur in the spleen and stomach. The treatment strategy is "acute convulsion is treated by cooling and purging, and chronic convulsions are treated by warming and supplementing." This strategy has been followed by physicians since then. When convulsions are acute they belongs to patterns of heat, yang and repletion; chronic ones happen slowly and they belong to patterns of cold, yin and vacuity.

Acute Convulsion

Etiology and Pathology

Acute convulsion happens fast and abruptly, there is a high fever, accompanied with convulsion and coma, it is mainly caused by exterior wind or warm pestilence. The location of it is in the liver and heart.

The exogenous evils invading The lungs in childhood are particularly delicate, their skin is tender and Wei Qi is weak. They also are not able to change their clothes according to the weather, so children are easily invaded by exterior wind. Wind is the leading causative factor of many diseases, it has the characters of constant movement and tends to transform into heat. If wind heat changes into wind, the children's liver and heart might be disturbed because of their weak mind, this is why they easily have convulsion due to high fever.

The warm pestilent toxin invading The epidemic toxin lingers in the body during warm febrile diseases, such as measles, pneumonia, mumps, and dysentery due to damp toxin. The heat toxin invades the heart and Ying level which results in convulsion and coma.

Being frightened suddenly Because of the weak mind and spirit, the children are easily frightened by seeing strange and horrible images, or hearing a strong voice, or suddenly falling down. The fright leads to disorder of qi and phlegm retention due to the qi disorder, disturbs the clear orifices, resulting in convulsion and coma.

Diagnosis

Diagnostic Guidelines

There is a history of invasion of exterior pathogens or warm febrile diseases The symptoms come on suddenly, in addition there are the manifestations of syndromes of phlegm, fever, scared and wind.

Differentiation of Diagnosis

Convulsions are different from epilepsy. Epilepsy often happens in older children who have repeated episodes without fever. When it attacks, there is an animal-like sound in throat, seizure, foaming at the mouth, accompanied by incontinence of urine and bowl movement. EEG shows waves consistent with epileptic wave patterns.

Diagnostic Notes

- Convulsions are related to the age of the patient. Physicians need to ask the patient's age. They must also ask if the convulsions are accompanied with fever, triggers of convulsions, and how long the convulsions last.
- Note the season at the time time of onset and characteristics of infectious diseases. Check the particular signs of the

nervous system and pathological reflexes that help make a diagnose.

- It is helpful for physicians to know the severity of the convulsions. Note changes in consciousness, pupil reactivity, respiration, heart rate, pulse rate, blood pressure, note changes in the anterior fontanel and muscle tension.
- The earlier the better to order the following labs: CBC, CMP, urine and stool routine examinations, calcium, magnesium, and other necessary medical tests. CSF, EEG, CT and MRI of the head all have significant diagnostic value.

Pattern Differentiation

Guidelines of pattern differentiation

The physician must differentiate between phlegm, heat, fright and wind, the four syndromes of convulsions. If there is a high fever, reddish face and eyes, thirst preferring cold water, constipation, and scanty urine, it is a heat pattern. If there is cough with copious phlegm, gargling in throat with unconsciousness or coma, it is a phlegm pattern. If there is anxiety, frightened with crying, restlessness and fear, it is the terrified pattern. If there is lockjaw, eyes staring, convulsion of extremities, stiffness of neck or even opisthotonos, it is the wind pattern. Some patients who have the convulsion syndrome may have the manifestations of phlegm, frighten, heat and wind together. Determine the severity of the convulsions. If the convulsions are less frequent and short in duration, it is considered a mild syndrome mostly due to wind-heat disturbing the liver. If the convulsions are frequent and repeat incessantly, or the convulsions stop but the patient is still unconscious, it is a critical convulsion syndrome due to severe toxin invading the Jueyin.

Therapeutic Principle

The main therapy is to clear the heart and resuscitate from unconsciousness, cool the liver and calm the wind. Clear heat, resolve phlegm and stop frighten according to the syndrome.

Patterns and Treatment

Convulsions due to exterior wind

Manifestations

Fever, cough, running nose, restlessness, convulsions, red tongue with thin yellow coating, wiry pulse or purple index vein.

Treatment Principle Clear heat and resolve exterior wind, calm the mind and extinguish wind.

Formula

Yin Qiao San (Honeysuckle and Forsythia Powder) modified.

Jin Yin Hua (Honeysuckle Flower) and Lian Qiao (Arid Forsythia Fruit) clear toxin and heat. Jing Jie (Schizonepeta), Bo He (Herba Menthae Haplocalycis) and Dan Dou Chi (Prepared Soybean) expel exterior wind. Niu Bang Zi (Arctium Fruit), Jie Geng (Platycodon Root), Dan Zhu Ye (Bamboo Leaf), Lu Gen (Rhizoma Phragmitis Communis) and Gan Cao (Licorice) expel wind-heat and soothe the throat. Add Chan Tui (Periostracum Cicadae), Gou Teng (Ramulus Cum Uncis Uncariae) and Shi Jue Ming (Concha Haliotidis) to expel wind and calm convulsions. If there is high fever with constipation, also add Liang Ge San (Cool the Diaphragm Powder). If the convulsions aer severe, you may also use Ling Jiao Gou Teng Tang (Antlope Horn and Uncaria Decoction).

Warm pestilent toxin invading

Interior enclosing of pestilent toxin

Manifestations

In addition to the manifestations of the original warm disease, there is high fever, anxiety, thirst, sudden convulsions of the extremities, staring eyes, unconsciousness and coma, purple or dark face, cold extremities and hidden pulse, red tongue with yellow greasy coating, or deep and purple index vein at the Ming (life) gate.

Treatment Principle Cool the liver, calm wind, clear the heart and open the orifices.

Formula

Ling Jiao Gou Teng Tang (Antlope Horn and Uncaria Decoction) and Zi Xue Dan (Purple Snow Special Pill)

Ling Yang Jiao (Cornu Antelopis), Gou Teng (Ramulus Cum Uncis Uncariae), Chuan Bei Mu (Bulbus Fritillariae Cirrhosae), Ju Hua (Flos Chrysanthemi Morifolii), Sang Ye (Folium Mori Albae), Bai Shao (Radix Paeoniae Lactiflorae) and Sheng Di Huang (Radix Rehmanniae Glutinosae) clear heat and cool blood, cool the liver and calm wind. Zi Xue Dan (Purple Snow Special Pill) clears heat, relieves toxicity, and opens orifices. If there is high fever, add Zhi Zi (Fructus Gardeniae Jasminoidis) and Huang Qin (Radix Scutellariae Baicalensis) to clear heat and toxicity. If there is coma and sever irritability, add An Gong Niu Huang Wan (Calm the Palace Pill with Cattle Gallstone) to clear heat and open orifices. If there is phlegm, add Shi Chang Pu (Rhizoma Acori Graminei), Tian Zhu Huang (Bambusa Textilis) and Dan Nan Xing (Arisaemae Cun Felle Bovis) to expel phlegm and open the orifices. If there are frequent convulsions add Quan Xie (Buthus Martensi) and Di Long (Lumbricus) to stop the wind.

Severe fire in qi and ying level

Manifestations

Sudden intense fever, severe and stabbing headache, delirious speech, coma, frigid extremities, rashes, raspy breathing, red tongue with yellow greasy coating, rapid pulse, or deep purple index vein at Ming gate

Treatment Principle Clear qi and cool the Ying level, calm the wind and open the orifices

Formula

Qing Wen Bai Du Yin (Clear Epidemics and Overcome Toxin Decoction)

In the formula, Shi Gao (Gypsum) and Zhi Mu (Rhizome Anemarrhenae) clear heat in the Qi level.

Huang Qin (Radix Scutellariae Baicalensis), Mu Dan Pi (Cortex Moutan Radicis), Sheng Di Huang (Radix Rehmanniae), Zhi Zi (Fructus Gardeniae Jasminoidis) and Chi Shao (Radix Paeoniae Rubra) clear heat and toxicity, cool the blood and quicken the blood. If there is unconsciousness or coma and convulsions, add Zi Xue Dan (Purple Snow Special Pill) or An Gong Niu Huang Wan (Calm the Palace Pill with Cattle Gallstone) or Zhi Bao Dan (Greatest Treasure Special Pill).

Damp-heat pestilent toxin

Manifestations

Intense high fever, frequent convulsions, delirious speech, severe irritability, abdominal pain, vomiting, pus in the feces, red tongue with yellow greasy coating, slippery and rapid pulse.

Treatment Principle Clear heat and eliminate dampness, relieve toxin and calm wind

Formula

Huang Lian Jie Du Tang (Coptis Detoxicating Decoction)

In the formula, Huang Lian (Rhizoma Coptidis), Huang Qin (Radix Scutellariae Baicalensis) and Zhi Zi (Fructus Gardeniae Jasminoidis) clear heat and relieve toxin. Add Ling Yang Jiao (Cornu Antelopis), Gou Teng (Ramulus Cum Uncis Uncariae) to calm wind and relieve convulsions. If there are sluggish bowel movements, add Da Huang (Radix et Rhizoma Rhei) and Hou Po (Cortex Magnoliae

Officinalis) to clear heat stagnation in the large intestine. If there are severe convulsions and coma, add Zi Xue Dan (Purple Snow Special Pill) or An Gong Niu Huang Wan (Calm the Palace Pill with Cattle Gallstone) or Zhi Bao Dan (Greatest Treasure Special Pill) to clear heat, open orifices and calm wind.

Being frightened suddenly

Manifestations

Sudden onset, sudden convulsion after being frightened, unconsciousness, anxiety, complexion with blue or changes to red or white, cold extremities, knotted pulse.

Treatment Principle Calm the liver and suppress mind.

Formula

Hu Po Bao Long Wan(Amber Holding Dragon Pill)
   In the formula, Hu Po (Amber) and Gou Teng (Ramulus Cum Uncis Uncariae) calm the frightened mind. Tian Zhu Huang (Bambusa Textilis) and Dan Nan Xing (Arisaemae Cun Felle Bovis) expel phlegm and open the orifices.

Other Treatment

Patent herbs

- Xia Er Hui Chun Dan (Return of Spring for Children Pill) It clears heat, arrests spasms and convulsion, transforms phlegm. The dosage is one pill taken 2~3 times daily under one year of age. Two pills taken 2~3 times from one to two years of age. It is used for convulsions due to exterior wind.
- Xiao Er Niu Huang San(Pediatric Cattle Gallstone Powder) It clears heat and calms fright and convulsions. The dosage is 0.3g~0.5g taken 2 times daily under one year of age. 0.9g

taken 2 times from two to three years of age. It is used for all acute convulsions.

Acupuncture

Du26, LI4, PC6, Liv3, Ki1, Yintang for convulsion. Du14, Shixuan (bleeding) for high fever. Add St40 if there is lot phlegm in the throat. Add St7 and St6 if there is lockjaw. All of the points are strongly stimulated.

Ear acupuncture

Strongly stimulate Ear Shenmen, and subcortical.

Strongly press Du26 with tip of thumb for waking up the patient from unconsciousness.

Prevention and care

- If the child has a fever, and especially for those with previous history of convulsion, pay particular attention to reduce their fever. Utilize therapies that include physical cooling, acupuncture, herbs, Tuina and medicine according to the specific condition of the patient.
- Put the child in the lateral recumbent position, move away any objects that may harm them. put the tongue wrapped with gauze between the upper and lower teeth to prevent biting the tongue if the child has onset of convulsions.
- If a seizure occurs while the patient is in clinic, it is recommended to call 911.

Chronic Convulsion

Etiology and Pathology

Chronic convulsions are mostly caused by chronic diarrhea, vomiting, or long term severe sickness.

Spleen yang vacuity It is often due to acute and chronic diarrhea, vomiting or incorrect treatment to promote sweating and purging, which damages the spleen yang, and the spleen fails to produce blood, the heart mind and liver wood are insufficiently nourished, resulting in interior wind.

Spleen and kidney yang vacuity This is due to chronic diarrhea, or improper/untimely treatment of spleen yang vacuity which develops into yang vacuity of spleen and kidney, leading to vacuity of Qi, blood, essence and body fluid. These multiple vacuities fail to nourish the heart and liver.

Wind stirring due to yin vacuity This is due to the protracted course of warm diseases or after acute convulsion, which causes heat to linger inside the body, or other chronic damage to the kidney yin, the water of kidney fails to nourish wood, resulting chronic convulsions.

In summary, the chronic version is caused by vacuity of spleen yang or spleen and kidney yang, which leads to qi and blood vacuity; heat damages the yin or kidney yin vacuity fails to nourish the heart and liver. The location of the disease is in the spleen, kidney, heart and liver. Most of these patterns are vacuous. If the patient has a red complexion, red lips and tongue, thin and rapid pulse, it is due to yin vacuity.

Therapeutic Principle

The main treatment is to supplement. Then address accompanying symptoms by nourishing the heart and opening the orifices, nourishing the liver and extinguishing wind. Warming and supplementing the spleen yang if there is spleen yang vacuity. Warm the spleen and kidney if there is yang vacuity of spleen and kidney. Nourish yin and blood if there is wind stirring due to yin vacuity.

Patterns and Treatment

Spleen yang vacuity

Manifestations

Pale complexion, drowsiness and fatigue without spirit, dim consciousness, occasional twitching or trembling, watery and loose stool, pale tongue with white and greasy coating, thread pulse.

Treatment Principle Warm and supplement the spleen yang, soften the liver and extinguish wind.

Formula

Huan Gan Li Pi Tang (Soft the Liver and Regular Spleen Decoction)
In the formula, Dang Shen (Radix Codonopsitis Pilosulae), Gan Cao (Radix Glycyrrhizae) and Bai Zhu (Rhizoma Atractylodis) strengthen the spleen and stomach. Bai Shao (Radix Paeoniae Lactiflorae) and Gou Teng (Ramulus Cum Uncis Uncariae) soften the liver and calm wind. If there is spleen vacuity affecting kidney yang that fails to warm the spleen, and the patient also has very pale complexion without any brightness, also add Fu Zi (Radix Aconiti Carmichaeli) and Rou Gui (Cortex Cinnamomi Cassiae) to warm the spleen and kidney yang.

Spleen and kidney yang vacuity

Manifestations

Very pale complexion, drowsiness and fatigue without spirit, dim consciousness, twitching, cold extremities with cold sweating, watery diarrhea, pale tongue with slippery coating, very deep and weak pulse.

Treatment Principle Warm the spleen and kidney yang, astringe yang and expel cold.

Formula

Gu Zhen Tang (Stabilize the True Decoction)

In the formula, Ren Shen (Radix Ginseng) strongly supplement Yuan qi, Fu Zi (Radix Aconiti Carmichaeli) and Rou Gui (Cortex Cinnamomi Cassiae) warm the fire of Ming Men. Huang Qi (Radix Astragali Membranaceus), Bai Zhu (Rhizoma Atractylodis), Fu Ling (Sclerotium Poria Cocos), Shan Yao (Radix Dioscoreae Oppositae) and Gan Cao (Licorice) supplement spleen qi. If there are frequent convulsions, shallow breathing, and redness around the zygomatic arch and hidden pulse, also add Long Gu (Os Draconis) and Mu Li (Concha Ostreae) to calm yang and rescue collapse.

Wind stirring due to yin vacuity

Manifestations

Low grade fever, emaciation, hot and twitching limbs, constipation, red tongue with dry and less coating, thin and wiry pulse.

Treatment principle Nourish yin and subdue yang, calm wind and stop convulsion.

Formula

Da Ding Feng Zhu(Precious Decoction for Ceasing Wind).

In the formula, Bai Shao (Radix Paeoniae Lactiflorae) and Sheng Di Huang (Radix Rehmanniae Glutinosae), Mai Men Dong (Tuber Ophiopogonis Japonici) and E Jiao (Colla Corii Asini) nourish Yin and ease the liver. Gui Ban(Plastrum Testudinis), Mu Li (Concha Ostreae) and Bie Jia (Carapax Testudinis) nourish Yin and subdue liver Yang. Wu Wei Zi (Fructus Schisandrae Chunensis), Zhi Gan Cao (Honey-fried Radix Glycyrrhizae Uralensis) produce yin with their sweet and sour nature. If there is obvious low grade fever, also add Yin Chai Hu (Radix Stellariae), Mu Dan Pi(Cortex Moutan Radicis) and Di Gu Pi (Cortex Lycii Radicis) to clear vacuous heat. If there is stiffness of limbs, also add Quan Xie (Buthus Martensi), Di Long (Lumbricus) and Wu Gong(Scolopendra Subspinipes) to expel wind and stop convulsions.

Other Treatment

Patent herbs

- Shu Huo Xiang Wan
- Xiao Er Hu Po Wan

Acupuncture

Strongly stimulate Du26, PC6, LI11, LI4, UB57, Liv3 and St7.
Moxa Du14, UB20, UB23, Ren3, Ren6, Du20 and St36. This is used for spleen yang or spleen and kidney yang vacuity.

Tuina

Push and knead spleen earth, transform interior Bagua, Divide yin and yang, push upper three gates, knead Ki 1 and St36. 5 to 15 minutes for each point, once every day.

Prevention and care

- Prevent injury to joints and muscles by avoiding strong pulls.
- Frequently change posture of the patient. Sponge baths using a soft towel with warm water, rub pressure areas or with alcohol to circulate Qi and blood and prevent bed sores.
- Frequently clean the mouth, nasal cavity.

Epilepsy (Xian Zheng痫证)

Epilepsy is also locally named as goat epileptic wind. It is a paroxysmal mental disorder, manifested with sudden collapse, loss of consciousness, staring upward, convulsions of limbs, spitting of white and frothy saliva or making a noise like a goat. Between epilepsy attacks, there is an interval, at which the patient looks healthy. It may also show a transient disturbance of consciousness or behavioral abnormalities. Epilepsy was recorded in the *Classic TCM of Yellow Emperor on the Strange Diseases,* but physicians had mixed the convulsion and epilepsy, until Qian Yi in the Song dynasty, in his book, *Xiao Er Yao Zheng Zhi Yue* (Key to Differentiation and Treatment of Disease of Children) mentioned that there are five kinds of epilepsy. The prevalence of epilepsy in children is about 3 ~ 6 %, occurring at any age. The sick children with frequent attacks usually have retarded intelligence.

Etiology and Pathology

Epilepsy during childhood is related to severe disturbance to the fetus during pregnancy, convulsions, wind, phlegm and poor early childhood nutrition.

Congenital factors If the pregnant mother hasn't been cared for correctly, it leads to Qi disorder and effects the development of the fetus. This especially causes disorders of the heart, liver, spleen and kidney, which easily generates wind and phlegm resulting in susceptibility to epilepsy.

Acquired factors Acquired factors may trigger onset of epilepsy.

- Epilepsy due to depression and terror: The child's brain function is physiologically insufficient. If a child has long term depression or is frightened suddenly, Qi is disordered and the mind is disturbed which causes wind and phlegm to cloud the heart orifice, resulting in epilepsy.
- Epilepsy due to phlegm: Incorrect diet may damage the spleen and stomach, which generates phlegm and clouds the heart, giving rise to sudden mental cloudiness and epilepsy.
- Epilepsy due to blood stasis: If the child is injured by birth trauma or falling down, the the blood vessels are damaged. Blood stasis stays in the brain and stagnates the heart orifice, and epilepsy occurs.
- Epilepsy due to repeated episodes of convulsion: If there are repeated episodes of acute or chronic convulsions, the wind and phlegm stagnate in the brain and mind, clouding the heart spirit and will results in epilepsy.

In general, wind and phlegm are direct factors of epilepsy. The main pathology is wind and phlegm misting upwards, blocking the heart orifice, and liver wind stirring up. The root causes of epilepsy are vacuities of the zang fu, disorders of qi, wind and phlegm deeply hidden in body. Since the interior phlegm mainly relates to spleen and kidney, the locations of epilepsy are at the heart, liver, spleen and kidney. The wind has characteristics of easy activation and motility, and phlegm has features of accumulation and spreading, therefore, the epilepsy occurs intermittently.

Diagnosis

Diagnostic Guidelines

- There is a history of similar episodes
- The common manifestations are sudden collapse, loss of consciousness, staring upward, convulsions of the limbs, spitting of white frothy saliva or making a noise like a goat. Between epileptic attacks, there are intervals in which the patient looks healthy. There may also be a transient disturbance of consciousness, abnormal behavior, headache, abdominal pain
- There is history of birth trauma, head trauma, or convulsion due to high fever
- Epilepsy can be confirmed through EEG study

Differential Diagnosis

Febrile convulsions are different from epilepsy. They occur at the beginning of a cold or flu with high fever. Children who are 6 months to 3 years old can easily have it. During each course of the disease, the convulsions will typically only happen once.

Diagnostic Notes

- Obtain a detailed history, such as if there is a history of birth trauma or asphyxia.

- All patients should be given an EEG.
- It is necessary for some of cases to perform topographical study of the brain or brain CT scan.

Pattern Differentiation

Guidelines of differentiation

Differentiate the severity If the onset is of short duration, episodes are intermittent with long intervals in between and twitching is light, it is a mild case. If seizures are frequent, there are frequent and sudden collapses, foaming at the mouth, gurgling in the throat, limbs twitching, incontinence of urination and feces, it is a severe case. If the convulsions don't cease on their own, it is critical.

Differentiate between wind, phlegm, terrified and blood stasis If the main symptom is convulsion, it is epilepsy due to wind. If there is unconsciousness, or even coma with a lot phlegm in throat, it is epilepsy due to phlegm. If there is a history that the patient was frightened, and the patient has anxiety, fears and is easy to be startled, it is epilepsy due to terror. If the patient has a history of injury or trauma, it is epilepsy due to blood stasis.

Therapeutic Principle

If it is in the attack stage, the main treatment is to strongly eliminate phlegm, extinguish wind, calm fright and open the orifice. If it is in the remission stage, treat the root and secondary syndromes.

Patterns and treatment

Epilepsy due to wind

Manifestations

Sudden onset and collapse, loss of consciousness, blue complexion, staring upward, lockjaw, convulsion of limbs, spitting of saliva, rigidity of the neck, thick and greasy coating, wiry pulse, or purple index vein.

Treatment Principle Extinguish wind, relieve convulsion, open orifice and calm spirit.

Formula

Ding Xian Wan (Stopping Epilepsy Pill)
In the formula, Tian Ma (Rhizoma gastrodiae elatae) and Quan Xie (Buthus martensi) calm the liver and expel wind. Chuan Bei Mu (Bulbus fritillariae cirrhosae), Zhu Li (Succus bambuae), Shi Chang Pu (Rhizoma Acori Graminei) and Ban Xia (Rhizoma Pinelliae Ternae) eliminate phlegm and open orifice. Fu Po (Succinum), Fu Ling (Sclerotium poria cocos) and Yuan Zhi (Radix polygalae tenuifoliae) anchor the heart and settle the mind. Dan Shen (Radix Salviae Miltiorrhizae) quickens the blood, Mai Men Dong (Ophiopogon root) nourishes yin. If the patient has anxiety and irritability due to excessive fire of the heart, also add Huang Lian (Rhizoma Coptidis) and Dan Zhu Ye(Herba lophatheri). If there is headache, dizziness and short temper, add Ju Hua (Flos Chrysanthemi Morifolii) and Chuan Xiong (Radix Ligustici Chuanxiong). If there are frequent convulsions, also add Ling Yang Jiao (Antelope Horn) and Gou Teng (Ramulus Cum Uncis Uncariae).

Epilepsy due to phlegm

Manifestations

Sudden collapse, unconsciousness, phlegm gurgling in throat, copious frothy saliva in the mouth, white and greasy coating, wiry and slippery pulse

Treatment Principle Strongly relieve phlegm and open orifice.

Formula

Di Tan Wan (Strongly Relieve Phlegm Pill)
In the formula, Ban Xia (Rhizoma Pinelliae Ternae), Chen Pi (Pericarpium Citri Reticulatae) and Tian Nan Xing (Prepared Arisaema Consanguineum with Bile) dry dampness and relieve phlegm. Zhi Shi

(Fructus Immaturus Citri Aurantii) and Zhu Ru (Tangand Bamboo Shavings) eliminate phlegm, regulate Qi and open the chest. Shi Chang Pu (Rhizoma Acori Graminei) opens the orifice and wakes up the mind. Ren Shen (Radix Ginseng), Fu Ling (Sclerotium Poria Cocos) and Gan Cao (Licorice Root) strengthen the spleen and relieve phlegm. If there is anxiety and fullness of the chest, add Huang Lian (Rhizoma Coptidis) and Yu Jin (Tuber Curcumae). If there is constipation, add Da Huang (Radix et Rhizoma Rhei, rhubarb).

Epilepsy due to Fear

Manifestations

After the patient has a severe cry, fear, anxiety, sudden red or pale or purple complexion, the patient could have a sudden attack of seizures and unconsciousness, green and sticky feces, red tongue, wiry and irregular pulse.

Treatment Principle Nourish heart and calm the mind, resolve phlegm and relieve fear.

Formula

Ding Po Wan (Calm Soul Pill)
     In the formula, Fu Shen (Poria Spirit), Yuan Zhi (Radix Polygalae Tenuifoliae), Suan Zao Ren (Semen Zizyphi Spinosae) and Fu Po (Succinum) nourish the heart yin and calm the mind. Deng Xin Cao (Juncos Effusus) clears heart fire. Ren Shen (Radix Ginseng) and Tian Men Dong (Tuber Ophiopogonis Japonici) supplement Qi and nourish yin. Tian Ma (Rhizoma Gastrodiae Elatae) and Shi Chang Pu (Rhizoma Acori Graminei) extinguish wind and open orifice.

Epilepsy due to Blood stasis

Manifestations

Sudden onset and collapse, loss of consciousness, convulsion of limbs with headache that is a stabbing and fixed pain, purple complexion, lips and tongue, choppy pulse. The patient often has trauma before having seizure.

Treatment Principle Remove blood stasis, open the orifice and stop seizure.

Formula

Tong Qiao Huo Xue Tang (Unblock the Orifices and Invigorate the Blood Decoction)

In the formula, Tao Ren (Semen Persicae), Hong Hua (Flos Carthami Tinctorii), Chi Shao (Radix Paeoniae Rubra) and Chuang Xiong (Radix Ligustici Chuanxiong) promote circulation and remove stasis. She Xiang (Secretio Moschus) unblocks the brain and opens the orifice. Sheng Jiang (Rhizoma Zingiberis Officinalis Recens) and Da Zao (Fructus Zizphi Jujubae) regulate Ying and Wei. Add. Ling Yang Jiao (Antilope Horn) and Gou Teng(Ramulus Cum Uncis Uncariae) to anchor fear and stop convulsions. If there is qi stagnation, add Qing Pi (Pericarpium Citri Reticulatae Viride) and Zhi Shi (Fructus Immaturus Citri Aurantii).

Other Treatment

Patent herbs

- Niu Huang Qing Xin Wan(Cattle Gallstone Pill to Clear Heart). It clears the heart, relieves phlegm, extinguishes wind and calm the mind. The dosage is 1/5 pill taken one time daily under five years of age.
- Fu Po Bao Long Wan (Succinum Holding Dragon Pill). It anchors fear, calms the mind, relieves phlegm and opens the orifice. One pill taken, twice daily.

Acupuncture

During attack: Du26, Ki1, LI4, PC6, and Du20. Use reducing technique, do not retain the needles.

During remission: Du14, UB15, Ht7, St40, Sp36 and GB20. Use even method, do not retain the needles.

Prevention and care

- Prevent trauma of birth and others.
- Be cautious with the diet, try to stay away from fatty, fried and spicy food, avoid overeating.
- Avoid overstress, and be careful of medications that have side effects for children.
- Be careful of accidents when the ill patient has frequent seizures.
- Pay attention to keep the airway open. Suction and oxygen maybe necessary during an epileptic attack.
- During an attack place the patient in a comfortable position. Move away any furniture that they may strike or fall into. Do not restrain or hold the patient tightly. Do not place anything in their mouth.

Attention Deficit Hyperactivity Disorder (Zhu Yi Li Que Xian Duo Dong Zheng 注意力缺陷多动症)

Attention-Deficit/Hyperactivity Disorder (ADHD) is characterized primarily by inattention, easily distracted, disorganization, procrastination, and forgetfulness; where it differs is in lethargy/fatigue, and having fewer or no symptoms of hyperactivity or impulsiveness typical of the other ADHD subtypes. Different countries have used different ways of diagnosing ADHD. Current estimates suggest that ADHD is present throughout the world in about 1~5% of the population. The American Psychiatric Association states in the Diagnostic and Statistical Manual of Mental Disorders (DSM-IV-TR) that 3~7% of school-aged children have ADHD (http://www.cdc.gov/ncbddd/adhd/data.html). About five times more boys than girls are diagnosed with ADHD. There is no record in ancient Chinese literature, but according to the manifestations of the disease, such as inattention, easily distracted, disorganization, procrastination, forgetfulness, anxiety and other clinical manifestations these are similar to the syndrome of "Zang Zao" or "forgetfulness" in Traditional Chinese Medicine.

Etiology and Pathology

Children who have congenital and acquired insufficiency, imbalance between Yin and Yang of the Zang Fu, or Yin failing to control Yang, this can result in inattention and easy distraction.

Hyperactivity of Liver Yang due to Kidney vacuity If a child has congenital vacuity that causes kidney yin insufficiency, the water fails to nourish the wood, resulting in hyperactivity of liver Yang and therefore, the inattention occurs.

Insufficiency of the heart and spleen If Yin and Qi vacuity fail to nourish the heart, the mind can't work cooperatively, thereby, a child becomes easily distracted. The spleen tends to stillness, stores Yi (ability to think and remember) and is in charge of thinking. If the spleen and heart are vacuous, the children's spirit will be uncertain, resulting in forgetfulness.

Phlegm fire disturbing the heart Damp-heat accumulation in the body turns to phlegm, phlegm heat disturbs the heart-mind, which also results in hyperactivity and inattention.

Moreover, blood stasis due to birth trauma, traumatic brain injury and fall injury blocking the brain orifice, also results in ADD/ADHD.

In summary, the causes of this syndrome are due to an imbalance between yin and yang, excessive yang activity, and insufficient yin stillness. It is caused by congenital vacuity, improper diet, or the Zang Fu organs are damaged. The root of the disease is vacuity of the spleen and kidney. The branch is excessive fire of the heart and liver. The location is at the heart, spleen, liver and kidney.

Diagnosis

Diagnostic Guidelines

These guidelines are according current ICD 10 criteria. (http://www.who.int/classifications/icd/en/GRNBOOK.pdf)

At least six of the following symptoms of attention have persisted for at least six months, to a degree that is maladaptive and inconsistent with the developmental level of the child:

G1 Inattention

(1) Often fails to give close attention to details, or makes careless errors in school work, work or other activities;
(2) Often fails to sustain attention in tasks or play activities;
(3) Often appears not to listen to what is being said to him or her;
(4) Often fails to follow through on instructions or to finish school work, chores, or duties in the workplace (not because of oppositional behavior or failure to understand instructions);
(5) Is often impaired in organizing tasks and activities;
(6) Often avoids or strongly dislikes tasks, such as homework, that require sustained mental effort;
(7) Often loses things necessary for certain tasks and activities, such as school assignments, pencils, books, toys or tools;
(8) Is often easily distracted by external stimuli;
(9) Is often forgetful in the course of daily activities.

G2 Hyperactivity

At least three of the following symptoms of hyperactivity have persisted for at least six months, to a degree that is maladaptive and inconsistent with the developmental level of the child:

(1) Often fidgets with hands or feet or squirms on seat;
(2) Lleaves seat in classroom or in other situations in which remaining seated is expected;
(3) Often runs about or climbs excessively in situations in which it is inappropriate (in adolescents or adults, only feelings of restlessness may be present);
(4) Is often unduly noisy in playing or has difficulty in engaging quietly in leisure activities;
(5) Exhibits a persistent pattern of excessive motor activity that is not substantially modified by social context or demands.

G3 Impulsivity

At least one of the following symptoms of impulsivity has persisted for at least six months, to a degree that is maladaptive and inconsistent with the developmental level of the child:

(1) Often blurts out answers before questions have been completed;
(2) Often fails to wait in lines or await turns in games or group situations;
(3) Often interrupts or intrudes on others (eg butts into others' conversations or games);
(4) Often talks excessively without appropriate response to social constraints.

Differentiation of Diagnosis

Tourette syndrome It is an inherited neuropsychiatric disorder with the onset in childhood, characterized by multiple physical (motor) tics and at least one vocal (phonic) tic. These tics characteristically wax and wane, can be suppressed temporarily, and are preceded by a premonitory urge. Tourette's is defined as part of a spectrum of tic disorders, which includes provisional, transient and persistent (chronic) tics.

Mental retardation The child has some of the same manifestations of ADD/ADHD, but they also have lower intelligent quotient and other symptoms of mental retardation.

Diagnostic Notes

- Note that this disease is mainly based on a continuous record of the assessment of children's behavior-based on the parents and kindergarten teachers.
- Note the onset age of the disease, the child has restlessness sleep usually at an early age. The symptoms become more

evident when they are in kindergarten, preschool or primary school.

- Attention can be tested if necessary.

Pattern Differentiation

Guidelines of differentiation

Differentiation of zang fu If there is anxiety, irritability, lack of cooperative, impulsivity, hyperactivity and restlessness, it is a syndrome of the liver. If there is fatigue, easily distracted, poor memory, pale nails and hair, it is a syndrome of the kidneys. If there is anxiety and night mare, it is a syndrome of the heart. If there is fatigue and weakness, restless thinking, it is a disorder of the spleen.

Differentiation of repletion and vacuity It is often a syndrome of repletion and vacuity. There may be concomitant hyperactivity of liver Yang and kidney vacuity, vacuity of heart and kidney, vacuity of spleen and heart. There are also repletion syndromes, such as fire phlegm disturbing the heart and blood stasis blocking interior.

Therapeutic Principle

Regulating zang fu and balancing yin and yang are the principles, also combining education and behavioral therapy.

Patterns and treatment

Hyperactivity of liver yang due to kidney vacuity

Manifestations

Inattention, anxiety, irritability, impulsivity, stubborn, hyperactivity, talkative, emaciation, red cheeks, nails and hair without luster, five center hot sensation, thirsty, prefer to drink cold water, red tongue with little fluid, wiry and rapid pulse.

Treatment Principle Nourish liver and kidney, anchor yang and stop the hyperactivity

Formula:

Qi Ju Di Huang Wan (Lycium fruit, chrysanthemum, and rehmannia pill)

In the formula, Mu Dan Pi (Cortex Moutan Radicis), Fu Ling (Sclerotium Poria Cocos), Shan Yao (Radix Dioscoreae Oppositae), Shan Zhu Yu (Fructus Corni Officinalis), Shu Di Huang (Radix Rehmanniae Glutinosae Conquitae) and Ze Xie (Rhizoma Alismatis Orientalis) are ingredients of Liu Wei Di Huang Wan (Six-ingredient Pill with Rehmannia) and nourish kidney Yin. Ju Hua (Flos Chrysanthemi Morifolii) clears liver heat, Gou Qi Zi (Fructus Lycii) nourishes liver and kidney yin. If there is obvious hyperactivity of liver Yang, also add Gui Ban (Plastrum Testudinis) and Mu Li (Concha Ostreae). If there is fire flaring upwards of Ming Men, also add Zhi Mu (Rhizome Anemarrhenae) and Huang Bai (Cotex Phellodendri).

Vacuity of the spleen and heart

Manifestations

Pale and dull complexion, emaciation, tired, easy distractibility, poor memory, pale and swollen tongue with thin white coating, deep weak pulse.

Treatment Principle Nourish the heart and strengthen spleen, calm the mind and stop hyperactivity.

Formula

Gui Pi Tang (Restore the Spleen Decoction) and Gan Mai Da Zao Tang (Glycyrrhizae Whaet and Jujubae Decoction)

The Gui Pi Tang guides the mind to the heart and spleen, Gan Mai Da Zao Tang helps the Zang Zao. If there is insomnia, add He Huan Pi (Cortex Albizziae Julibrissin), Ye Jiao Teng (Caulis

Polygoni Multiflori) and Long Gu (Os Draconis). If there is forgetfulness, add Shi Chang Pu (Rhizoma Acori Graminei).

Phlegm fire disturbing the heart

Manifestations

Hyperactivity, hyper talkative, short temper, easily angered, easily distracted, inattention, a lot phlegm and bitter taste in mouth, yellow urine, red tongue with yellow greasy coating, slippery and rapid pulse.

Treatment Principle: clear heat and resolve phlegm, calm the heart mind.

Formula: Huang Lian Wen Dan Tang (Coptidis Warm the Gallblader Decoction)

In the formula, Huang Lian(Rhizoma Coptidis), Ban Xia (Rhizoma Pinelliae Ternatae) and Zhu Ru (Phyllostachys Nigra) clear heat and calm the mind, dry dampness and resolve phlegm. Chen Pi (Pericarpium Citri Reticulatae) regulates Qi, Fu Ling (Sclerotium Poria Cocos) strengthens spleen and eliminates phlegm. All the ingredients clear heat, resolve phlegm and calm the heart-mind. If there is constipation, add Da Huang (Radix et Rhizoma Rhei) to purge heat in Fu organs. If there is a bitter taste in the mouth and yellow urine, add Zhi Zi (Fructus Gardeniae Jasminoidis) to clear heat and expel anxiety.

Acupuncture

Acupuncture points: Du20, Si Shen Chong, Du14, Du24, UB15, Du4, PC6, and LI11. Use purging treatment without needle retention. Once a day, 7~10 day is a course of treatment.

Ear needles: Ht, Shen Men, Jiao Gan(Sympathetic), brain stem, subcortex, kidney. Puncture superficially without retention. Once a day, 7~10 day is a course of treatment. Place seeds on your selection of the above ear points twice in a week, alternate ears every time. Press each point for one minute, three times per day. Complete three courses of treatment.

Prevention and care

- Pay attention to the nutrition, nursing and education of the fetus during pregnancy. Avoid premature delivery, dystocia and suffocation.
- Prevent the injury of brain and poison. Actively prevent disorders and infections of central nervous system.
- Note mental health of children, prevent negative stimulus of psychological, keep quiet and intimate living and learning environment.
- Reasonable arrangements for rest, training a regular life.

Viral Myocarditis in Children (Xiao Er Bing Du Xing Xin Ji Yan 小儿病毒性心肌炎)

Pediatric myocarditis is inflammation of the heart muscle in an infant or young child. In children it is usually caused by viruses that reach the heart, such as the influenza (flu) virus, Coxsackie virus, parovirus, and adenovirus. However, it may also be caused by bacterial infections, including Lyme disease. The symptoms may be mild at first and hard to detect. However, in newborns and infants, symptoms may sometimes appear suddenly. It is manifested with fever, fatigue, pale complexion, palpitations, shortness of breath, cold extremities and sweating. It usually occurs after flu, diarrhea and mumps. Children may have it during any seasons. It tends to be more severe in newborns and young infants than in children over age 2. An acute myocardial infarction-like syndrome with normal coronary arteries has a good prognosis; severe cases may lead to vacuity of heart yang, exhaustion of heart yang, or even death. Some cases may become chronic due to incorrect treatment diet, or no treatment.

It relates to wind and febrile-warm diseases, palpitations and chest Bi within the context of Chinese medicine. The primary

195

pathogens are usually wind, heat and damp toxin, accumulation of heat toxin, which leads to injuring qi an yin of the heart. In addition, overwork, depression or long-term stress may be triggers. Heat invading the heart after wind, heat and damp toxins invade the body, accumulate in the lung and stomach, excessive heat toxin damages the qi and yin, resulting in disorders of the heart circulation manifesting as myocarditis.

Etiology and Pathology

Vacuity of both qi and yin of the heart If heat toxin lingers inside, and consumes qi and yin or the patient hasn't been cared for correctly, the qi and yin is further damaged. Therefore, the qi and yin fails to nourish the heart, resulting in symptoms of myocarditis.

Heart yang vacuity In this case the patient hasn't been treated in time, or correctly and the progress of the disease will lead to heart yang vacuity. The yang is then too weak to warm and circulate the heart and vessels, resulting in exhaustion of heart yang, and becomes critical.

Concomitant phlegm and blood stasis If a child has insufficient lung, spleen and kidney qi, all of them easily tend to dampness and phlegm which affects the circulation of the heart, resulting in phlegm mixing with blood stasis in the chest. Therefore, the patient might have some of the symptoms of myocarditis, such as distress of chest and palpitations.

Qi vacuity with evils lingering When the patient suffers long term and the evils still lingers inside, along with weakened Vital Qi, the weak qi will become even weaker, and the evils lodge deeper in the body.

In summary, the main pathology of the disorder is heat in the heart with Qi and Yin vacuity, and blood stagnates in the vessels.

Diagnosis

Diagnostic Guidelines

- Previously, the patient had an infectious disease, such as flu, diarrhea, mumps, or German measles.

- There are manifestations of heart failure, cardiogenic shock, fatigue, pale and dull complexion, palpitations, shortness of breath, fullness of chest, sighing, cold extremities, aching muscles, rapid pulse, or knotted pulse.
- The Electrocardiogram(ECG) and serum creatine phosphokinase and serum lactic dehydrogenase may help the diagnosis.

Diagnostic Notes

- Be sure to inquire if the patient has a history of infectious disease before the onset of the current symptoms.
- There are not any typical manifestations in infants, but they might have cyanosis, cold extremities, staring eyes and poor appetite.
- Carefully do auscultation on the heart to know the sound, rates, rhythm of heart.

Pattern Differentiation

Guidelines of differentiation

Severity If the patient has few symptoms and a strong pulse, it is a mild syndrome. If the patient has anxiety, pale complexion, purple lips and deep, weak pulse, or knotted, intermittent pulse, it is a severe case.

Differentiation of repletion and vacuity If the patient has a short history of sickness accompanied by heat in the lungs and stomach, it is considered a replete pattern If the patient has a long history of sickness accompanied with fatigue, pale and dull complexion, palpitation, shortness of breath and pale tongue, it is considered a vacuity pattern.

Therapeutic Principle

Supplement the heart qi and nourish heart yin, remove blood stasis and unblock vessels is the primary treatment principle. If there is evil toxin invading the heart, also clear heat and resolve toxin. If there is heart yang vacuity you must rescue the heart yang. If there is mixing of the phlegm and blood stasis, add medicinals to strongly expel phlegm and remove blood stasis.

Patterns and Treatment

Heat invading the heart

Manifestations

Palpitations, shortness of breath, chest pain and fullness of chest, aching body; accompanied with runny nose, chills and fever, cough, sore throat, red tongue with thin and yellow coating, floating rapid pulse

Treatment Principle Clear heat, resolve toxin, calm the heart and regulate the pulse.

Formula

Yin Qiao San (Honeysuckle and Forsythia Powder) modified.

This formula clears heat and expels exterior syndromes, resolves toxin and soothes the throat. If the heat is excessive, add Huang Qin (Radix Scutellariae Baicalensis), Zhi Zi (Fructus Gardeniae Jasminoidis) and Shi Gao (Gypsum) to clear heat and purge fire. If there is fullness of chest, add Yu Jin (Tuber Curcumae) and Mu Xiang (radix Aucklandiae Lappae) to regulate qi and open the chest. If there is chest pain, add Hong Hua (flos Carthami Tinctorii) and Dan Shen (Radix Salviae Miltiorrhizae) to remove blood stasis. If there is severe sore throat, add Shan Dou Gen (Ophora Subprotrata), Ban Lan Gen (Radix Isatidis Seu Baphicacanthi) and Xuan Shen (Radix Scrophulariae Ningpoensis) to expel toxin and soothe the throat. If there is a greasy tongue coating, or fullness of chest, add Gua Lou (Fructus Trichosanthis), Ban Xia (Rhizoma Pinelliae Ternae) and Yu Jin (Tuber Curcumae) to drain damp and clear heat.

Vacuity of both qi and yin of the heart

Manifestations

Palpitations, anxiety, fullness of chest and shortness of breath, fatigue, insomnia, spontaneous or night sweating, pale or red tongue body with less coating, thin and knotted pulse.

Treatment Principle Supplement qi, nourish yin, calm the heart and regulate pulse.

Formula

Sheng Mai San (Generate the Pulse Powder)
　　Ren Shen(Radix Ginseng), Mai Men Dong(Tuber Ophiopogonis Japonici) and Wu Wei Zi (Fructus Schisandrae Chinensis) supplement qi and nourish Yin of the heart. If qi vacuity is especially evident, add Huang Qi (Radix Astragali Membranaceus) to supplement qi. If yin vacuity is more obvious, add Sheng Di Huang (Radix Rehmanniae Glutinosae) and Yu Zhu (Rhizoma Polygonti Odorati) to nourish Yin. If there are palpitations and restlessness, add Ye Jiao Teng (Caulis Polygoni Multiflori) and Suan Zao Ren (Semen Zizyphi Spinosae) to calm the mind. If there is pale complexion, fatigue, and a pulse is severe knotted, add Zhi Gan Cao Tang (Honey-fried licorice Decoction) to nourish the heart.

Heart yang vacuity

Manifestations

Dizziness, palpitations, fatigue, cold extremities, spontaneous sweating, purple lips and nails, pale and purple tongue, thin and white tongue coating, deep and thin pulse

Treatment Principle Warm heart yang.

Formula

Gui Zhi Gan Cao Long Gu Mu Li Tang (Cinnamon Twig Decoction Plus Dragon Bone and Oyster Shell)

Gui Zhi (Ramulus Cinnamomi Cassiae) and Gan Cao (Radix Glycyrrhizae) warm the heart Yang. Long Gu (Os Draconis) and Mu Li (Concha Ostreae) calm the mind and stop sweating. If fatigue and weakness are severe, add Huang Qi (Radix Astragali Membranaceus) and Ren Shen (Radix Ginseng) to supplement Qi. If there is severely cold extremities, add Fu Zi (Radix Aconiti Lateralis Praeparata) and Gan Jiang (Rhizoma Zingiberis) to warm Yang and expel cold.

Mixing of phlegm and blood stasis

Manifestations

Palpitations, shortness of breath, fullness and pain of the chest, cough with copious phlegm, pale and purple tongue with white and greasy coating, choppy or knotted pulse.

Treatment Principle Eliminate phlegm, calm the heart, remove blood stasis.

Formula

Gua Lou Xie Bai Ban Xia tang (Trichosanthes Macrosterm and Pinellia Decoction) and Shi Xiao San (Sudden Smile Powder)

Gua Lou Xie Bai Ban Xia Tang (Trichosanthes Macrosterm and Pinellia Decoction) eliminates phlegm, opens the chest, unblocks vessels and stops pain. Shi Xiao San (Sudden Smile Powder) removes blood stasis and stops pain. If there is phlegm heat, add Huang Qin (Radix Scutellariae Baicalensis) and Zhu Ru (Phyllostachys Nigra) to clear heat and resolve phlegm. If blood stasis is severe, add Hong Hua (flos Carthami Tinctorii) and Dan Shen (Radix Salviae Miltiorrhizae). If there is restlessness during the night, add Bai Zi Ren (Semen biotae orientalis) and Ye Jiao Teng (Caulis Polygoni Multiflori) to nourish the heart and calm the mind. If there is severe sweating, add Long Gu (Os Draconis) and Mu Li (Concha Ostreae) to stop sweating.

Qi vacuity with evils lingering

Manifestations

Pale and dull complexion, tired, palpitations, shortness of breath, sighing poor appetite, spontaneous sweating, easy to get sick, sore throat, pale tongue with white coating, sluggish pulse or knotted pulse.

Treatment Principle Strengthen Qi to expel pathogens, nourish Yin and regulate pulse.

Formula

Huang Qi Gui Zhi Wu Wu Tang (Astragalus and Cinnamon Twig Five-Substance Decoction).

Huang Qi (Radix Astragali Membranaceus) supplements Qi and strengthens Wei Qi, Gui Zhi (Ramulus Cinnamomi Cassiae) and Bai Shao (Radix Paeoniae Lactiflorae) harmonize the Ying and Wei, warm and unblock the heart Yang. Sheng Jiang (Rhizoma Zingiberis Officinalis Recens) and Da Zao (Fructus Zizphi Jujubae) warm the middle and supplement vacuity. Yi Tang (Saccharum Granorum) supplements the vacuity of the middle Jiao. Gan Cao (Radix Glycyrrhizae Uralensis) harmonizes all functions of the herbs. If the palpitations are obvious, add Long Gu (Os Draconis) and Mu Li (Concha Ostreae) to calm the mind of heart. If there is anxiety and poor sleep, add Wu Wei Zi (Fructus Schisandrae Chunensis) and Suan Zao Ren (Semen Zizyphi Spinosae) to nourish the heart and calm the mind. If the patient is susceptible to catching colds, add Yu Ping Feng San (Jade Windscreen Powder) to supplement Qi and fortify the exterior. If there is a sore throat, add Shan Dou Gen (Ophora Subprotrata), Ban Lan Gen (Radix Isatidis Seu Baphicacanthi) to relieve toxin and soothe the throat.

Other Treatment

Patent herbs

- Sheng Mai Yin (Generate the pulse Liquid) This formula can supplement Qi, regulate the pulse, nourish Yin and generate fluids. It is used for Qi and Yin vacuity patterns. Taken orally 5~10 cc/time, 2~3 times per day.
- Fu Fang Dan Shen Pian (Compound Salvia Pill) This formula can remove blood stasis, regulate Qi and stop pain. It is used for chest pain due to blood stasis. Taken orally 1~2 pill/time, 2~3 times/day.

Prevention and care

- Make sure to get enough rest and avoid strong physical exertion to prevent re-occurrence
- Avoid exposure to large groups of people
- Dress appropriately for the weather
- Take measures to avoid catching infectious diseases as these may trigger this disease

Diseases and Syndromes of Kidney

The kidneys are located at the level of the waist, they store essence and they metabolize water. The essence stored in the kidney is the foundation of development, growth and the overall proper functioning of the Zangfu organs. The kidney is the root of acquired qi. Disorders such as edema, enuresis, frequent urination, and proteinuria may all be related to water metabolism and are all considered disorders of the kidney. The common pathology of these disorders is a breakdown of the Qi Hua function. They are also related to the transformation and transportation function of the spleen and the descending and downbearing function of the lungs. This means that normal fluid metabolism depends on the cooperation of the lung, spleen and kidney. Exterior pathogens easily attack the lung during childhood, which triggers the edema or makes it worse. The spleen's primary function is the transformation and transportation of food and fluids; it is referred to as Yun Hua in Chinese. The spleen's Yun Hua function relies heavily on the kidneys Qi Hua function while the kidney relies on the spleen for supplementation. When there is chronic spleen vacuity, it will lead to kidney vacuity. A dual vacuity of spleen and kidney is very common. Supplementing the spleen and kidney is a common practice and will be discussed later. The liver stores blood and is the wood phase; the kidney stores essence and is the water phase. The essence can generate blood and the blood can transform into essence. This is why it is said that the liver and kidney have the same source. If the kidney essence fails to nourish liver wood, there may be dual vacuity of liver and kidney yin.

Chronic disorders may enter the Luo Channels, leading to blood stasis and ultimately water retention. In the clinic, the edema may easily cause qi stagnation and blood stasis.

Enuresis (Yi Niao 遗尿)

A child who is older than 5 and continues to wet the bed at night is considered to have enuresis. There is a primary and secondary type of enuresis. The primary type is the more common type in the clinic. It is related to family history. Incidence of enuresis is more prevalent in males than female by up to 3:1. Most of the primary enuresis cases are due to functional disorders. Secondary enuresis is often accompanied by systemic or renal system disorders.

Etiology and Pathology

The production of urine is related to the water metabolic function of the lung, spleen and kidney.

Kidney yang vacuity When a child is born congenitally weak, this will lead to Kidney yang vacuity. Therefore the urinary bladder will not function properly due to the kidney qi failing to regulate the urinary bladder.

Spleen and lung vacuity The lungs govern qi. The lungs are the upper source of water. The lungs control the function of descending water to the urinary bladder. The spleen is the earth phase, and controls the transformation and transportation of food and fluids. If the lung Qi is too weak to descend water into the urinary bladder or the spleen qi is too weak to ascend water up to the lungs, there may be enuresis.

Damp-heat in the liver meridian The liver soothes and regulates the qi. If dampness and heat accumulate in the liver meridian, it will disrupt the smooth flow of qi and allow the dampness and heat to accumulate in the lower Jiao. This causes disorders of the urinary bladder, including enuresis.

Diagnosis

Diagnostic Guidelines

- The child must be over 5 years old.
- There is bedwetting one or more times per night during sleep. They sleep deeply and are difficult to wake up.
- No abnormalities are found in routine urinary examinations.

Diagnostic Notes

- Inquire if there is frequent, painful, scanty and urgent urination. These may indicate a Lin syndrome pattern.
- Ask the parents about daily urinary patterns. Ask about toilet training methods and progress.
- Observe the constitution of the child, examine the genital area looking for eczema, redness or swelling
- Differentiate between other diseases that cause bedwetting such as Xiao Ke, lower IQ, urinary tract deformation, and pinworms.

Pattern Differentiation

- Urinary Incontinence Urine spontaneously leaks, day or night, awake or asleep. This disorder often has multi-system accompanying symptoms.
- Heat Lin Syndrome This refers to frequent, painful and scanty urination. The standard urinary test indicates RBC and WBC in the urine as well as bacteria present in the urine culture.

Guidelines of differentiation

Focus on differentiation between cold and heat, vacuity and repletion of the Zang Fu organ systems. Differentiate between the syndromes of kidney yang vacuity, vacuity of lung and spleen and damp-heat in the liver meridian according to the course of illness, urinary frequency, volume, smell and accompanying symptoms.

Therapeutic Principle

The main principle is supplementing qi for patterns of vacuity, such as warming the kidney and restoring essence, supplementing the lung and spleen, and clearing heat and draining dampness from the liver. In addition, clearing the heart, unblocking the heart orifice and awakening the mind might be added for the other cases.

Patterns and treatment

Kidney yang vacuity

Manifestations

Bed wetting once or more every night, profuse and clear urine, fatigue, pale face, cold extremities, weak lower back and legs, pale tongue, deep and weak pulse.

Treatment Principle Warm the kidney yang, stop enuresis

Formula

Tu Si Zi San (Cuscuta Seed Pill)

In the formula, Tu Si Zi (Semen Cusecutae Chinensis), Rou Cong Rong (Herba Cistanches Deserticolae), and Fu Zi (Radix Aconiti Lateralis Praeparata) warm kidney yang and benefit the lower Jiao. Wu Wei Zi (Fructus Schisandrae Chinensis) and Mu Li (Concha Ostreae) strengthen kidney and prevent bed wetting. If there is oversleep and cloudiness due to phlegm accumulation, add Shi Chang Pu (Rhizoma Acori Graminei) and Yuan Zhi (Radix Polygalae Tenuifoliae) to resolve phlegm and open orifices. If there is poor appetite and loose stool, add Si Jun Zi Tang (Four Gentle Man Decoction) to transform and transport fluids.

Lung and spleen vacuity

Manifestations

Bed wetting once or more every night, frequent urination during the day, susceptibility to cold, cough, shortness of breath, spontaneous sweating, pale face, poor appetite, loose stool, pale tongue with white coating, deep and weak pulse.

Treatment principle Supplement the lung and strengthen spleen, stop enuresis

Formula

Suo Quan Wan (Shut the Sluice Pill) and Bu Zhong Yi Qi Tang (Tonify the Middle and Augment the Qi dection)
   In the formula, Ren Shen (Radix Ginseng), Bai Zhu (Rhizoma Atractylodis), Huang Qin (Radix Scutellariae Baicalensis), Sheng Ma (Rhizoma Cimicifugae), Chai Hu (Radix Bupleuri) strengthens spleen qi. Dang Gui (Radix Angelicae Sinensis) and Zhi Gan Cao (Honey-fried Radix Glycyrrhizae Uralensis) supplement qi and blood. Yi Zhi Ren (Fructus Aliniae Oxyphyllae), Wu Yao (Radix Linderae Strychnifoliae) and Shan Yao (Radix Dioscoreae Oppositae) strengthen kidney qi and astringe fluids. If there is a desire to sleep and difficulty waking up, add Shi Chang Pu (Rhizoma Acori Graminei) to open the heart orifice. If there is loose stool add Pao Jiang (Quik-fried Rhizoma Zingiberis) to warm spleen yang.

Damp heat in liver meridian

Manifestations

Bed wetting, scanty and yellow urine, short temper, dream disturbed sleep, teeth grinding during sleep, 5 palm burning sensation, red complexion, red lips, red eyes, thirsty with desire to drink, red tongue with yellow coating, wiry and slippery pulse.

Treatment principle Clear heat and eliminate dampness, prevent leakage.

Formula

Bi Quan Wan(Secreting Urination Decoction)
In the formula, Bai Shao (Radix Paeoniae Lactiflorae) soothes and softens the liver, Zhi Zi (Fructus Gardeniae Jasminoidis) clears heat, Bai Zhu (Rhizoma Atractylodis) strengthens the spleen, Bai Lian (Radix Ampelopsis) and Yi Zhi Ren (Fructus Aliniae Oxyphyllae) astringes the urine. If there is yellow greasy tongue coating, add Huang Bai (Cortex Phellodendri) to clear damp-heat. If there is kidney Yin vacuity, add Zhi Bai Di Huang Wan (Anemarrhena, Phellodendron, and Rehmannia pill) to nourish Yin and extinguish fire. If there is a red tongue with scanty coating, add Shi Hu (Dendrobium Stem) and Shan Yao (Radix Dioscoreae Oppositae).

Other Treatment

Patent herbs

- Sang Piao Xiao San (Mantis Egg-case Powder) is used for bed wetting due to the dual vacuity of heart and kidney. Taken orally 3~6g 2 times per day.
- Jin Suo Gu Jing Wan (Metal Lock Pill to Stabilize the Essence) is used for bed wetting due to kidney vacuity. Taken orally 3~6g, 2 times per day.
- Long Dan Xie Gan Tang(Gentian Liver-Purging Decoction) is used for damp-heat stagnation in the liver meridian. Taken orally 3~6g, 2 times per day.

Acupuncture

Ren 3, Ren 6, Sp 6, Sp 9, St 36, Yin Tang. Choose 2~3 points per treatment. The extra point, Yi Niao Xue (Bed Wetting point) it is located on the palmar surface of the little finger, in the middle of the transverse crease of the distal interphalangeal joint.

Ear points: Kidney, UB, subcortex, Shenmen, endocrine, lung, spleen.

Moxibustion at Ren 8, Sp8, 20 minutes for vacuity pattern.

Tui Na

Knead Ren 6 for 200 times. Rub Du 4, Ba Liao, each for 20 minutes.

Herbs for Topical Use

Ground 3g of Wu Bei Zi (Gallnut of Chinese Sumac) into a powder. Mix it with warm water, then put it on the umbilicus, and cover with a bandage. Place it before putting the child to bed. Do this once a day for 3-5 days is a course of treatment.

Adjunctive Care

- When children have enuresis, no scolding, no irony and no punishment. Try to build confidence and reduce their burden.
- Adhere to bladder training and proper control of drinks before bedtime. Encourage urination before bedtime. Each night the child should be awakened to urinate, this can train the children to wake up before wetting the bed.

Prevention and care

- Create a good family atmosphere. Develop good habits and avoid excessive stress and fatigue. Avoid having soup and water after dinner.
- Empty the bladder as much as possible before going to sleep. Replace wet sheets in time. Avoid over-excitement, and avoid incorrect urinary habits. Patiently educate and guide the child. As the child progresses be sure to encourage them.

Pediatric Heat Lin Syndrome
(Xiao Er Re Lin小儿热淋)

Heat Lin means frequent and urgent urination, a sub-type of Lin syndrome. *Dan Xi Xing Fa*, (The New Method of Dan Xi) 1481 said: "Lin means dripping and scanty urine, belonging to a heat syndrome." The *Zhu Bing Yuan Huo Lun* (General Treatise on the Causes and symptoms of diseases) 610 stated: "frequent urination is due to heat accumulating in the urinary bladder and kidney". Infants have a high incidence; the incidence of females is 3 to 4 times more than boys. Most urinary tract infections belong to the pattern of heat Lin.

Etiology and Pathology

Heat Lin is commonly caused by damp heat in the urinary bladder and impairment of qi transformation.

Damp heat in the lower Jiao A girl's urethra is short and the external orifice of the urethra is exposed, therefore it is easily invaded. There are several mechanisms which may lead to damp-heat accumulation including: urinary accumulation at the prepuce (also referred to as the clitoral hood), constipation, and over-holding of urine leading to the urinary bladder becoming over-filled. All of these lead to heat Lin due to damp toxin easily invading the urinary bladder and impairment of Qi transformation.

Damp-heat accumulation due to qi vacuity of spleen and kidney
Spleen qi vacuity diminishes the ascending of clear qi, and transformation of fluids. Kidney qi vacuity impairs qi transformation, which leads to damp-heat lingering, resulting in a chronic condition. If the protracted course of disease consumes the Yang of the spleen and kidney, it allows pathogens to easily invade the body and the syndrome often reoccurs. The dampness and heat linger in the body and damage yin, leading to a mixed syndrome of yin vacuity and damp-heat stagnation. The prolonged course of this syndrome may also be due to an abnormal urinary tract formation.

In Summary, heat Lin syndrome is located in the kidney and urinary bladder, and dampness and heat are the main pathogens. The damp-heat accumulation in the urinary bladder is a repletion pattern. Spleen and kidney vacuity with damp-heat in the urinary bladder is a mixed syndrome of repletion and vacuity.

Diagnosis

Diagnostic Guidelines

Typical symptoms: A new born baby may have fever, vomiting, diarrhea, restlessness, but frequent and urgent urine is not so obvious. Infants and toddlers have obvious symptoms of the whole body with mild local symptoms. They may have fever, vomiting and diarrhea, interrupted urination, crying during urination, bed wetting, strong smelling urine, there may be intractable diaper rash, and erythema at the perineum. Preschool children have frequent, urgent, and painful urination accompanied with soreness of the back. Urinary laboratory tests may show leukocytes. Urine culture may have bacterial growth.

Diagnostic Notes

- Note that Heat Lin has special manifestations at different ages.
- Heat Lin in newborns is often associated with bacteremia. Inquire as whether or not the child is experiencing convulsions and observe for jaundice.
- Pay close attention to a newborn or toddler's urinary habits. Be aware of enuresis, strong smelling urine or interrupted urination. The genital and perineal area should be observed for intractable diaper rash, and erythema.
- Routinely check the child's urine if you suspect heat Lin syndrome. If it is a protracted course, urinary tract malformation is likely and relevant laboratory exams need to be done.

Pattern Differentiation

Guidelines of differentiation

Focus on identifying repletion and vacuity. If there is a sudden onset of symptoms, a short history, frequent, urgent, painful, and cloudy urination, hematuria, fever and chills, red tongue with yellow greasy coating, and a purple index vein it is a repletion pattern. If there is uneasy urination without pain, fatigue, pale tongue and pale index vein, it is vacuity with repletion.

Stone Lin manifests as scanty urination, interrupted urination, hematuria, visible or occult stones in the urine. X-ray or B-ultrasound can indicate positive findings.

Therapeutic Principle

In a repletion pattern, focus on clearing heat and draining dampness. If there is heat accumulation in the spleen and stomach, add herbs to activate the Fu organs and descend the qi. If there is heat in the liver and gall bladder, clear the liver and purge fire and toxins from the gall bladder. For mixed syndrome of repletion and vacuity supplement qi and kidney

Patterns and treatment

Damp-heat in the Urinary bladder

Manifestations

Sudden onset, frequent, burning, scanty and cloudy urine, lower abdominal distention, frequent crying. Accompanied with fever, thirst, anxiety, nausea, vomiting, red tongue with yellow and greasy coating, purple index vein.

Treatment Principle Clear heat and drain dampness

Formula

Ba Zheng San (Eight-herb Powder for Rectification)

In the formula Tong Cao (Tetrapanax Papyriferus), Hua Shi (Talcum), Qu Mai (Herba Dianthi), Bian Xu (Herba Polygoni Avicularis), Zhi Z (Fructus Gardeniae Jasminoidis), Da Huang (Radix et Rhizoma Rhei) and Gan Cao (Radix Glycyrrhiae Uralensis) clear heat. If there is abdominal distention, add Chai Hu (Radix Bupleuri), Yan Hu Suo (Corydalis Yanhusuo) to soothe the liver and relieve stagnation. If there is scanty and painful urine, thirst, anxiety, a red tongue with a thin coating, it is due to heart fire transforming in the small intestine. Add Dao Chi San (Guide out the Red Powder) to clear heat from the heart. If there is interrupted and painful urine, it is often due to a stone in the urinary tract. Add Jin Qian Cao (Glechoma Longituba), Da Ji (Herba Crisii Japonici) and Bai Mao Gen (Rhizoma Imperatae Cylindricae) to clear heat, stop bleeding and expel the stone.

Vacuity of spleen and kidney with damp-heat lingering in the urinary bladder

Manifestations

Chronic and reoccurring symptoms, frequent urination, pale face, poor appetite, cold extremities, loose stools, puffy lips, pale tongue with thin and greasy coating, thready pulse.

Treatment Principle: supplement kidney qi

Formula

Suo Quan Wan (Stop well pill)

In the formula, Yi Zhi Ren (Fructus Aliniae Oxyphyllae) and Shan Yao (Radix Dioscoreae Oppositae) supplement kidney and strengthen spleen. Wu Yao (Radix Linderae) regulates qi and stops pain. Add Fu Ling (Sclerotium Poria Cocos) and Che Qian Zi (Plantago Asiatica) to drain dampness. If there are manifestations of kidney Yang vacuity, such as pale complexion, cold extremities, puffy legs, profuse urine, pale tongue and weak pulse you can use Jin Gui Shen Qi Wan (Kidney Qi Pill from the Golden Cabinet) or You Gui Wan (Restore the Right Pill) to warm kidney yang and promote urine. If there are manifestations of kidney yin vacuity, such as low grade fever, dry throat and lips, red tongue with slight greasy coating, thin and rapid pulse, use Zhi Bai Di Huang Wan (Anemarrhena, Phellodendron, and Rehmannia Pill) to nourish yin, clear heat and eliminate dampness.

Other Treatment

Patent herbs

- San Jin Pian (Three Golden Pills) is used for heat Lin due to the damp heat in the urinary bladder. Taken orally 2 pills 2 times/day.
- Long Dan Xie Gan Wan(Gentian Liver-Purging Pills) is used for heat Lin due to damp-heat in the lower Jiao. Taken orally 6~9g, 2 times/day.

Acupuncture

UB23, UB28 and ear kidney, 5 minutes each time, 5 treatments is one course.

Tuina

Knead Dantian 200 times and abdomen for 20 minutes. It is used especially for spleen and kidney vacuity.

Herbs for Topical Use

Jin Yin Hua (Flos Lonicerae Japonicae), Pu Gong Ying (Herba Taraxaci Mongolici Cum), Di Fu Zi (Kochia Scoparia) and Bai Bu (Radix Stemonae) 30g each, cook the all herbs and then soak in it for 30 minutes, once per day. It is used for frequent, urgent and painful urine.

Huang Bai (Cotex Phellodendri)15g, Ku Shen (Radix Sophorae Flavescentis) 15g, Tu Fu Ling (Smilax Glabra)10g and She Chuang Zi (Fructus Cnidii Monnieri) 10g, cook the all herbs, and then soak in it 30 minutes, once per day. It is used for damp-heat in the liver and gall bladder.

Prevention and Care

Take special care of the vulva with infants, wash the buttocks well after bowel movements. Change the diapers frequently and try to have a regular change of pants. Encourage the children to drink more water, or drink sodium bicarbonate in water to alkalize urine. Cultivate a habit of the children defecating and urinating at the same times during the day. Encourage children to defecate and urinate once they feel the need in order to prevent constipation or holding back of urine. Try to find abnormalities in the urinary tract early. If a pinworm is found in the urethra, it should be treated immediately. If the patient has a fever, their diet should be light and bland. Spicy foods also should be avoided.

Acute Glomerulonephritis (Ji Xing Shen Xiao Qiou Shen Yan 急性肾小球肾炎)

Acute glomerulonephritis (AGN) is active inflammation of the glomeruli. It is manifested mainly with edema, hematuria, proteinuria and hypertension. This classically occurs after an infection with the bacteria *Streptococcus pyogenes*. It is also called post-infectious glomerulonephritis. AGN is the primary cause of hospitalized children suffering from urinary symptoms. Peak occurrences are during the winter in children ages 5 to 10 years old, in children under 2 years of age it is rare. The ratio between male and female is about 2:1. It follows after an infection of the respiratory tract or skin infections. Most of them have a good prognosis.

Chinese medicine believes that if fluid is retained and overflows to the skin, head, face, chest and abdomen, it is an edema syndrome and it belong to the category of yang edema, or hematuria and vertigo syndromes.

Etiology and Pathology

AGN is commonly caused by wind-heat, damp-heat, toxin, and disharmony among the lung, spleen and kidney.

Exterior pathogens invading lung Wind-heat-damp toxin invades the lung, resulting in the failure to disperse and descend, and blocking the water way. This leads to edema. Water stays inside of the body and flows downwards to the lower Jiao. Over time, it will engender heat which may burns the vessels, resulting in hematuria.

Damp heat stagnation disturbing the three Jiao Damp-heat in the three Jiao involves the Jue Yin, resulting in dizziness and headache in mild conditions and convulsions in critical conditions. Damp-heat accumulating downwards towards the lower Jiao makes the hematuria worse. Damp-heat blocks the water way, resulting in scanty or no urine, which causes palpitations and shortness of breath due to the water abnormally moving upwards and attacking the heart and lungs.

Vacuity of lung and spleen The vital qi is deficient after the pathogens are gone, which manifests as a pale complexion, fatigue, poor appetite, profuse sweating and susceptibility to reoccurrence.

In Summary, the main pathological factors of AGN are wind, damp and heat toxins lingering in the lung, along with damp-heat stagnation obstructing the three jiao. The location is in the lung, spleen and kidney. If treatment is incorrect, AGN may become chronic due to the lingering of damp-heat.

Diagnosis

Diagnostic Guidelines

History: An infection is present before the onset of the edema. For example there may have been a respiratory infection one to two weeks prior, or a skin infection two to three weeks prior to the edema.

Manifestations

Scanty urine and edema that start from the upper body and moves downward. Initially there are puffy eyelids in the early morning, gradually the edema occurs in the whole body. It is not pitting edema. In severe cases, there is hydrothorax or ascites. Some cases have hematuria or microscopic hematuria and symptoms of hypertension, such as dizziness and headache. Severe cases may have heart failure, hypertensive encephalopathy and acute renal failure. Laboratory tests can show protein, red or white blood cells in the urine, C_3 is reduced, anti-streptolysin (an anti-body for a strain of streptococcus), and O (ASO) and ESR increased.

Differentiation of Diagnosis

- Viral nephritis The patient has a history of viral infection, manifested by hematuria, no obvious edema and hypertension, no C_3 reduced and ASO increased. The prognosis is better than for AGN.
- Chronic nephritis The patient has a long history of renal illness. Most of them have malnutrition, anemia, hypertension, a lot of protein in the urine and symptoms of renal failure.

Diagnostic notes

- First ask age and sex of patient, and in what season the disease occurs. Also focus your inquiry on the presence of an infectious disease, such as streptococcus tonsillitis or scarlet fever occurring before the onset of the edema.
- Be sure to identify if the edema is pitting edema or not, and if there is a relationship between the volume of urine and hypertension.
- Test the routine urine for ASO and C_3 levels.

Pattern Differentiation

Guidelines of differentiation

- Identify the characteristics of the edema
- If there is an acute onset with a short course of illness, the edema starts from the eye lids and gradually affects the whole body with no pitting edema, it is Yang edema.
- Identify the accompanying patterns. If the edema is accompanied with chills and fever, sore throat and cough, it is due to wind invading the upper Jiao and the lungs fail to disperse and descend, resulting in wind mixed with water. If there are sores with pus on the skin, it is due to damp heat lingering inside.
- Identify the complications If there is scanty urine, abdominal bloating, cough, shortness of breath with palpitations, the syndrome of water disturbing the lung and heart is highly considered. If there is unconsciousness, convulsions, stiffness of the neck, and rapid breathing, the syndrome of a pathogen involving the pericardium and Jue Yin should be considered. If there is no urine, vomitus with a strong odor, loose stool, nose bleeding, it is the syndrome of water toxin closed inside and exhaustion of spleen and kidney should be considered.

Therapeutic principle

A repletion pathogen is the main mechanism in this illness. The treatment principle is to reduce repletion through sweating, purging, eliminating and clearing. The common treatments are to clear heat and toxin, drain dampness, disperse the lungs, and expel pathogens. If there is spleen qi vacuity with pathogens lingering in the lungs, supplement qi, clear heat and drain dampness. Be aware of complications and deal with them as they arise.

Patterns and treatment

Common Syndrome

The mixture of wind and water

Manifestations

Edema first occurring at the eye lids, gradually moving to the extremities, even spreading to the chest and abdomen, no pitting edema, scanty and yellow urine with hematuria, accompanied with chills and fever, cough, aching body, reddish, swollen and painful tonsils, thin and white coating, and floating pulse.

Treatment principle Expel wind and promote urine.

Formula

Ma Huang Lian Qiao Chi Xiao Dou Tang (Ephedra, Forsythiae and Phaseolus Calcaratus Decoction)

Ma Huang (Herba Ephedra) disperses evils and promotes urine. Lian Qiao (Fructus Forsythiae Suspensae) clears heat and toxin. Chi Xiao Dou (Phaseolus Calcaratus) promotes urination and reduces edema. If there is severe exterior cold, add Qiang Huo (Rhizoma et Radix Notopterygii) and Fang Feng (Radix Saposhnikoviae) expel wind and release the exterior syndrome. If there is severe interior heat, add Shi Gao (Gypsum) clear heat. If hematuria is obvious, add Bai Mao Gen (Rhizoma Imperatae Cylidricae) and Xiao Ji (Herba Cephalanoplos) clear heat and stop bleeding. If there is a sore and swollen throat, add Ban Lan Gen (Radix Isatidis Seu Baphicacanthi) clear heat and soothe the throat. If the edema is more evident in the lower part of the body, add Da Fu Pi (Pericarpium Arecae Catechu) eliminate dampness and water.

Damp heat stagnation

Manifestations

Mild edema, scanty urine, hematuria, sores on the skin, red tongue with yellow coating, slippery and rapid pulse.

Treatment principle

Clear heat toxin and drain dampness.

Formula

Wu Wei Xiao Du Yin (Five Ingredient Decoction to Eliminate Toxin) and Wu Pi San (Five peel powder).

Jin Yin Hua (Honeysuckle Flower), Pu Gong Ying (Herbal Taraxaci Mongolici Cum Radice), Zi Hua Di Ding (Herba Cum Radice Violae Yedoensitis), Ye Ju Hua (Flos Chrysanthmi Indici) and Zi Bei Tian Kui(Herba Begoniae Fimbristipulatae) clear heat and toxin. Sang Bai Pi (Cortex Mori Albae Radicis), Sheng Jiang Pi (Rhizoma Zingiberis Officinalis Recens), Fu Ling Pi (Cortex Poriae Cocos), Chen Pi (Pericarpium Citri Reticulatae) and Da Fu Pi (Pericarpium Arecae Catechu) drain dampness and reduce the edema. If the edema is severe, add Tong Cao (Tetrapanax Papyriferus) and Che Qian Zi (Plantago Asiatica) to promote urination and reduce edema. If there are sores on the skin, add Ku Shen (Radix Sophorae Flavescentis) and Bai Xian Pi (Cortex Dictammi Dasycarpi) to drain dampness and clear toxin. If hematuria is obvious, add Da Ji (Herba Crisii Japonici), Xiao Ji (Herba Cephalanoplos), Mu Dan Pi (Cortex Moutan Radicis) to cool the blood and stop bleeding.

Qi vacuity of the lung and Spleen

Manifestations

During the recovery stage of long term of illness where there is mild edema, pale face, fatigue, spontaneous sweating, susceptibility, pale tongue with white coating, weak and sluggish pulse.

Treatment principle Strengthen spleen and supplement qi.

Formula

Shen Ling Bai Zhu San (Ginseng, Poria, and Atractylodes Macrocephala Powder) and Yu Ping Feng San (Jade Windscreen Powder).

Shen Ling Bai Zhu San (Ginseng, Poria, and Atractylodes Macrocephala Powder) strengthens the spleen and drains dampness. Yu Ping Feng San (Jade Windscreen Powder) supplements qi and strengthens the defensive qi. If the case is chronic and there is kidney Yin vacuity, such as red tongue with less coating, thin and rapid pulse, add Liu Wei Di Huang Wan (Six-ingredient Pill with Rehmannia) to nourish kidney Yin.

Complicating Syndromes

Water toxin disturbing the heart and lung

Manifestations

Scanty or no urine, puffiness of the whole body, cough, shortness of breath, anxiety, difficult lying down, purple lips and fingers, white and greasy coating, deep and weak pulse.

Treatment principle Purge the lung, expel water, warm Yang and strengthen qi

Formula

Ji Jiao Li Huang Wan (Stephaniae Semen Rhuber Pill) and Shen Fu Tang (Ginseng Aconiti Decoction)

In the formula, Ting Li Zi (lepidium Apetalum), Da Huang (Radix et Rhizoma Rhei) purge the lung and expel water. Jiaomu (Semen Zanthoxyli) and Han Fang Ji (Radix Stephaniae Tetrandrae) promote urine. Ren Shen (Radix Ginseng) and Fu Zi (Radix Aconiti Lateralis Praeparata) warm yang. If there are cold extremities and sweating, add Rou Gui (Cinnamon Bark), Long Gu

(Os Draconis) and Mu Li (Concha Ostreae) to warm yang and stop sweating. If there is less urine, add Gui Zhi (Ramulus Cinnamomi Cassiae) and Ze Xie (Rhizoma Alismatis Orientalis) to warm yang and expel water.

The syndrome of pathogen involving Jue Yin

Manifestations

In addition to the edema, the patient has headache, dizziness, blurry vision, anxiety, or even convulsion and unconsciousness, a red tongue with yellow coating, and a wiry pulse.

Treatment principle Purge fire, drain dampness, calm the liver yang.

Formula

Long Dan Xie Gan Tang (Gentian Liver-Purging Decoction) and Ling Yang Gou Teng Tang (Antelope Horn and Uncaria Decoction). Long Dan Xie Gan Tang (Gentian Liver-Purging Decoction) clears excessive heat from the liver. Ling Yang Jiao (Antelope Horn, Gou Teng (Uncaria) calm the liver and expel wind. Bai Shao (Radix Paeoniae Lactiflorae) and Dang Gui (Radix Angelicae Sinensis) nourish Yin and supplement blood. If there is vomiting, add Ban Xia (Pinellia Ternatae) and Tian Nan Xing (Arisaema Consanguineum) to expel phlegm.

Closed syndrome due to water toxin

Manifestations

Severe edema, scanty or no urine, dizziness, headache, nausea, vomiting, unconsciousness, greasy tongue coating and wiry pulse.

Treatment principle Open closed syndrome with the pungent herbs and descend with the bitter, expel turbid dampness and toxin

Formula

Wen Dan Tang (Warm the Gall Bladder Decoction) and Fu Zi Xie Xin Tang (Aconiti Decoction to Drain the Epigastrium) Da Huang (Radix Rhizoma Rhei), Huang Qin (Radix Scutellariae Baicalensis) and Huang Lian (Rhizoma Coptidis) clear toxin and eliminate turbid dampness. Fu Zi (Radix Aconiti Carmichaeli) warms Yang, Gan Jiang (Rhizoma Zingiberis) opens the closed syndrome and warms the middle. Chen Pi (Pericarpium Citri Reticulatae) and Ban Xia (Rhizoma Pinelliae Ternatae) dry dampness and eliminate pathogens. Zhu Ru (Phyllostachys Nigra) and Zhi Shi (Fructus Immaturus Citri Aurantii) clear the gall bladder and harmonize the stomach.

Other Treatment

Patent herbs

- Shen Ling Bai Zhu San (Ginseng, Poria, and Atractylodes Macrocephala Powder) Taken orally 3g, three times per day. It is used for Qi vacuity of the lung and spleen.
- Zhi Bai Di Huang Wan (Anemarrhena, Phellodendron, and Rehmannia Pill) Taken orally 3g, three times per day. It is used for the remission stage due to kidney Yin vacuity.

Acupuncture

UB13, Lu7, LI4, Sp9, Ren9, UB22. Reducing technique. If there is sore throat, add Lu11. If there is facial edema, add Du26. If blood pressure is high, add LI11, Liv 3.

EAr Point: kidney, spleen, urine bladder, sympathetic, adrenal gland, endocrine. 2~3 points for each time. Once per day, ten times is a course of treatment.

Tuina

During attack stage, calm liver, lung, stomach, spleen and small intestine meridians. Reduce six Fu organs. At the remission stage, calm liver meridian, supplement kidney and spleen meridians, kneads Er Mang (Two Houses) and clear small intestine.

Topical therapy

- Xiao Zhong Fang (Reduce Edema Formula) Grand Shi Gua Pi (Loofah Peel) 30g, Dong Gua Pi (Winter Melon Peel) 30g and Yu Mi Xu (Corn Silk) 30g. Put on the umbilicus and cover with a bandage once per day. This is used for the attack stage.
- Washing therapy Qiang Huo (Rhizoma Radix Notopterygii), Ma Huang (Herba Ephedra), Jing Jie (Herbs Seu Flos Schizonepetae Tenuifoliae), Fang Feng (Radix Ledebouriella Divaricatae), Cang zhu (Rhizoma Atractylodis), Chai Hu (Radix Bupleuri), Niu Bang Zi (Fructus Arctii), Zi Su Ye (Folium Perillae) and Cong Bai (Bulbus Allii Fistulosi) each 20g, decoct and wait for the temperature to reach 102F and take a bath in the herb decoction. Take the child out of the bath once they begin to sweat. Perform this once per day.

Food therapy

Limit salt intake, water and protein during attack stage. If there is edema and hypertension, recommend salt reduction. In severe cases, restrict taking salt daily 60 ~ 120mg/kg. If there is azotemia, take protein daily 0.5g/kg.

- Fang Feng Congee Cook Fang Feng(Radix Ledebouriella Divaricatae)15g, two pieces of Cong Bai (Bulbus Allii Fistulosi) with water 150 c. second, take the herbs out from the decoction, then add washed Geng Mi (Sticky rice)100g into the decoction. Cook about 30 minutes. Take it as a meal. It is used for wind edema.
- Li Yu Chi Xiao Dou Tang (Carp and Phaseolus Calcaratus) A carp fish 250g, and Chi Xiao Dou 50g. Cook them as a soup, and drink it. It is used for edema with damp heat lingering inside.

Prevention and Care

It is essential to prevent this disease from becoming a streptococcal infection. Treat the illnesses such as tonsillitis, scarlet fever, impetigo and skin boils. Routinely test the urine in 2 to 3 weeks after infections to detect abnormalities in time. In the first 2 weeks of onset, provide plenty of bed rest. Take the child out to do minor activities after the edema and hematuria disappear, and blood pressure normalizes. The child may go to school when the erythrocyte sedimentation rate is close to normal, but should avoid strenuous exercise.

Nephrotic Syndrome
(Shen Bing Zong He Zheng肾病综合征)

Nephrotic syndrome (NS) is characterized by an increase in the permeability of the capillary walls of the glomerulus leading to the presence of high levels of protein passing from the blood into the urine, low levels of protein in the blood (*hypoproteinemia* or*hypoalbuminemia*), ascites, and in some cases, edema. There may also be high cholesterol (*hyperlipidaemia* or *hyperlipemia*) and a predisposition for coagulation. Nephrotic syndrome makes up about 21% of hospitalized cases in the pediatric urology department and is the second highest incidence occurring in the department, which seconds to acute nephritis. The males have significantly higher incidence than the females, 3 to 5 years of age is the age of peak onset. NS can be treated as edema and kidney water category. Edema's characteristics are written in the Yellow Emperor's Classic of Traditional Chinese Medicine. "All the syndromes of edema and fullness caused by the wetness evil are pertaining to the spleen". The *Zhu Bing Yuan Huo Lun* (General Treatise on the Causes and symptoms of diseases) 610 by Chao Yuan-fang stated "Edema is due to spleen and kidney vacuity". Dr. Zhu Dan Xi (1481) divided the edema into yang edema and yin edema. Most of the NS cases are yin edema, manifested by severe puffiness, re-occurrence, vacuous and cold syndromes.

Etiology and Pathology

The insufficiency of the spleen and kidney is the interior cause of NS, exterior pathogen invading is the cause for NS re-occurring.

- *Spleen vacuity and damp retention* During childhood, the spleen is inherently insufficient., If dietary habits or treatment are incorrect, it causes food stagnation, turning into dampness, and accumulating in the middle Jiao. The dampness damages spleen Yang which fails to transform and transport, resulting in water retention and edema occurring.
- *Vacuity of spleen and kidney* The spleen is the root of postnatal Qi, and the source of Qi and blood production. If the spleen vacuity damages the kidneys, it results in water retention and edema due to both spleen and kidney vacuity.
- *Vacuity of liver and kidneys* If there is a failure to store kidney essence, it leads to vacuity of the liver and kidneys, yin vacuity due to the leaking out of Yin essence. If NS has been treated with the warming medicinals for a long time, the Yin will be damaged. Hyperactivity of Yang due to Yin vacuity may burn the vessels and result in hematuria.
- *Qi and blood stasis* Yang qi vacuity slows down blood circulation, the blood stasis may turn into water retention. Water retention also hampers circulation.

In summary, NS belongs to yin edema. It is located in the spleen and kidney, but it may also include patterns of vacuity and repletion together, therefore, the course of treatment may be longer.

Diagnosis

Diagnostic Guidelines

Simple NS

It occurs in young children, from ages 2 to 7 years old at the time of onset. If the case has the following four characteristics:

- Pproteinuria, duration more than 2 weeks, 24 hours total urinary protein more than 0.1g / kg or 0.05g / kg;
- low blood albumin disease: serum albumin less than 30g / L;
- Hyperlipidemia: blood cholesterol> 5.7 mmol / L;
- Edema, excess proteinuria and low blood albumin are more important for the diagnosis of NS.

Nephritic NS

If the patient has the above manifestations, and also has one of the following: hematuria, recurrent hypertension, persistent azotemia, and total serum or serum complement C_3 repeatedly decreased, it can be diagnosed as nephritic NS.

Differentiation of Diagnosis

Acute glomerulonephritis There is occasional proteinuria but when combined with the history of the disease, main manifestations, nature of edema, ASO, serum complement C_3, cholesterol and serum albumin can help the differentiation.

Purpura NS There is a hemorrhagic rash with joint and kidney damage. Hemorrhagic rashes are located in the distal extremities, buttocks, lower abdomen, around the ankle to the knee. Commonly they present with symmetrical distribution. Kidney damaged often occurs 4~8 weeks after the rash.

Diagnostic Notes

First ask how long the edema has been present, ask if it reoccurs or lingers, and if it is associated with any infection. Note the severity of edema, if there is ascites or pitting Test protein volume in the urine for 24 hours, test serum albumin and cholesterol. Note if there are any complications of NS, such as infection and electrolyte imbalance.

Pattern Differentiation

Identify the location of the edema. If it is more swollen in the lower part of body, accompanied with dampness, then the pattern primarily involves the spleen. If there is ascites and edema at the wrist accompanied by cold intolerance and loose stool, both spleen and kidney are involved. If the edema is more obvious in the face, and accompanied by respiratory symptoms, the lungs are also involved. Identify the volume of urine. In general, the smaller the amount of urine, the worse the edema will be. If the urine output is increased, it indicates the edema is subsiding.

Therapeutic Principle

The main principle is to supplement qi, strengthen the spleen, warm yang, promote urination, relieve edema. If the kidney disorder insults the liver causing a concurrent vacuity of liver and kidney, the treatment is to nourish the kidney and sedate liver yang.

Spleen vacuity with damp retention

Manifestations

Pitting edema all over the body, pale complexion, fatigue, chest and abdominal distention, poor appetite, loose stool, scanty urination, cold extremities, pale and swollen tongue with a slippery and white coating, a deep and weak pulse.

Treatment Principle Warm spleen yang, regulate qi, promote urination, relieve edema

Formula

Shi Pi Yin (Strengthen Spleen Decoction)
Fu Zi (Radix Aconiti Carmichaeli) warms the yang and promotes urination. Gan Jiang (Dried Rhizoma Zinggiberis Officinalis) warms the spleen yang and help promotes urination. Fu Ling (Sclerotium

Poria cocos) and Bai Zhu (Rhizoma Atractylodis) strengthen the spleen and eliminate dampness. Mu Gua (Chaenomeles Lagenaria) invigorates the spleen and eliminates dampness. Hou Po (Cortex Magnoliae), Mu Xiang (Radix Aucklandiae Lappae), Bing Lang (Semen Arecae Catechu), Cao Guo (Fructus Amomi Tsao-ko) regulate qi and eliminate dampness. Gan Cao (Radix Glycyrrhizae Uralensis), Sheng Jiang (Rhizoma Zingiberis Officinalis Recens) and Da Zao (Fructus Zizphi Jujubae) strengthen spleen and harmonize the middle. If there is severe qi vacuity, add Dang Shen (Radix Codonopsitis Pilosulae) and Huang Qi (Radix Astragali Membranaceus) to supplement the spleen qi. If there is scanty urine, take out Mu Gua and add add Wu Ling San San (Five-ingredient Powder with Poria).

Yang vacuity of the spleen and kidney

Manifestations

Severe, pitting edema all over the body, puffy eye-lids, ascites, pleural effusion, pale complexion, fatigue, cold extremities, poor appetite, cough, shortness of breath, difficulty lying down, pale and swollen tongue with slippery, white coating, deep and week pulse.

Treatment principle Warm the yang and promote urination.

Formula

Zhen Wu Tang(True Warrior Decoction)
    In the formula, Fu Zi (Radix Aconiti Carmichaeli) warms yang and promotes urination, Fu Ling (Sclerotium Poria Cocos) and Bai Zhu (Rhizoma Atractylodis) strengthen the spleen and eliminate dampness, Sheng Jiang (Rhizoma Zingiberis Officinalis Recens) expel cold and harmonize the middle. If there is spleen Qi vacuity, also add Dang Shen (Radix Codonopsitis Pilosulae) and Huang Qi (Radix Astragali Membranaceus) to strengthen the spleen Qi. If the dampness is severe, add Wu Ling San (Five Ingredient Powder with Poria) promote urination and reduce edema. If there is severe kidney

yang deficiency, add Rou Gui (Cinnamon Bark) and Ba Ji Tian (Radix Morindae Officinalis) to warm kidney yang. If there is diarrhea, add Pao Jiang (Quick-fried Rhisoma Zingberis Officinalis) and Bu Gu Zhi (Fructus Psoraleae) to warm the spleen and kidney yang.

Yin vacuity of liver and kidney

Manifestations

Five palm burning sensation, hot flashes, dizziness and headache, thirst, soreness of the lower back and knees, sweating and constipation, red tongue with less coating, thin and rapid pulse.

Treatment principle Nourish kidney yin, sedate liver yang

Formula

Zhi Bai Di Huang Wan (Anemarrhena, Phellodendron, and Rehmannia Pill)
In the formula, Zhi Mu (Rhizome Anemarrhenae), Di Huang (Radix Rehmanniae Glutinosae), Huang Bai (Cotex Phellodendri) and Mu Dan Pi (Cortex Moutan Radicis), Shan Zhu Yu (Fructus Corni Officinalis) nourish the kidney Yin and clear deficient heat, Shan Yao(Radix Dioscoreae Oppositae) and Fu Ling(Sclerotium Poria Cocos) strengthen spleen and eliminate dampness, Ze xie (Rhizoma Alismatis Orientalis) eliminates dampness. If there is damp heat, also add Che Qian Zi(Plantago Asiatica) and Zhi Zi(Fructus Gardeniae Jasminoidis) clear heat and eliminate dampness. If there is heat toxin with Yin deficiency, add Jin Yin Hua(Flos Lonicerae Japonicae), Pu Gong Ying(Herba Taraxaci Mongolici Cum) cleat heat and toxin.

Qi stagnation and blood stasis

Manifestations

Dull or dark complexion, stubborn edema or not severe edema, sore lower back, constant blood in urine, purple tongue, choppy pulse.

Treatment principle Invigorate blood.

Formula

Tao Hong Si Wu Tang(Four-Substance Decoction with Safflower and Peach)

In the formula, Shu Di Huang(Radix Rehmanniae Glutinosae Conquitae), Bai Shao(Radix Paeoniae Lactiflorae), Dang Gui(Radix Angelicae Sinensis) and Chuan Xiong(Radix Lgustici Chuanxiong) nourish the blood and invigorate blood, Tao Ren(Semen Persicae) and Hong Hua(Flos Carthami Tinctorii) remove blood stasis. If there is severe blood stasis, also add Qian Cao(Radix Rubiae Cordifoliae), San Leng (Rhizoma Sparganii) remove blood stasis. If blood in urine, add Pu Huang(Pollen Typhae), and Bai Ji(Rhizoma Bletillae Striatae). If there is qi vacuity, add Dang Shen(Radix Codonopsitis Pilosulae) and Huang Qi (Radix Astragali Membranaceus) strengthen the spleen qi.

If there are some complications of this disorder, such as skin sores, or flu, please refer to the related chapters.

Other Treatment

Patent herbs

- Lei Gong Teng Duo Dai Pian(Tripterygium Glycosides Pill) 1mg/kg per day, separately oral taking 2~3 times. Total 6~12 weeks as one course of treatment. The side effects are uncomfortable stomach and intestine, skin rashes, lower white blood cells.
- Liu Wei Di Huang Wan(Six-ingredient Pill with Rehmannia) Oral taking 3g, three times per day. It is used for kidney Yin deficiency.
- Jin Gui Shen Qi Wan(Kidney Qi Pill from the Golden Cabinet) Oral taking 3g, two times per day. It is used for kidney Yang deficiency.

Acupuncture

(1)UB23, UB21, Liv3, St36, Sp6, Ren6 and Ren9. Tonifying manipulation. Once every other day. Ten treatments is one course.

Ear points

Spleen, kidney, subcotex, adrenal and urinary bladder. Choose 2~3points for each time for 30 minutes. Every other day, ten treatments is a course.

Tui Na

Supplement kidney 3 minutes, soften Er Ma, Dan Tian, Ren8 and San Guan, each for 2 minutes. It is used for Yang deficiency of spleen and kidney. Sedate liver, tonify kidney, soften Er Ma and Sp6, each for two minutes.

Diet

For a general patient, less salt is recommended for 1~2g per day. No salt is recommended for severe cases that have edema or hypertension. Even if the patient has had edema for long time, it is not necessary for patient to have no salt, the patient need control the volume of water that is drank according to the volume of the patient's urine in one day. The intake of protein and calorie of the patient are recommended to be the same as the intake of other healthy children. If the patient has a lot protein in the urine, the intake of protein that is needed is 2g/kg per day.

Food therapy

- Cook one carp and Chi Xiao Dou (phaseolus calcaratus) 50g as soup. Take it as food.
- Cook Huang Qi (Radix Astragali Membranaceus) 50g with chicken as soup. Take it every day.

Prevention and Care

- Actively prevent respiratory diseases, particularly upper respiratory tract infections.
- Dental caries and chronic tonsillitis should be treated in time.
- In order to enhance immunity, do more outdoor activities, and have exposure to sunlight.
- Try to keep the patient's skin clean.

Infectious Diseases

Infectious diseases are considered to be the warm diseases in Chinese medicine. Most of them have specific pathogenic factors, such as being infectious, epidemic or seasonal. They also have similar pathological processes, such as the development of diseases following the syndrome of Wei, qi, Ying and blood. They also may have the syndrome of both Wei and qi, or both qi and Ying, even all the syndromes of Wei, qi, Ying and blood together. Most of them have similar manifestations, for example, acute onset and fast transformation. Most of them have fever and rashes. They may easily include bleeding symptoms due to heat disturbing the blood, wind syndromes due to heat flaring upward, and closing or collapse syndrome. They also may have yin consumption or qi and yin vacuity in the later stages. Therefore, it is necessary to make an accurate and early diagnosis, to treat promptly, to isolate the patients, and to reduce the incidence of spreading. To get a correct diagnosis, the unique diagnostic method of febrile warm diseases have to be noted, such as observation of the tongue and teeth, identification of fever, rashes, sweating, spirit and convulsions. The most common treatment methods are expelling exterior, clearing Qi, harmonizing, eliminating dampness, purging, clearing Ying, cooling blood, opening orifices, extinguishing wind, nourishing yin, strengthening qi, and rescuing the depleted. It is important to prevent febrile diseases. Strictly isolate the source(s) of infection, and follow reporting guidelines according to the city's policy. Vaccination is also a key measure to prevent febrile diseases in children.

Measles (Ma Zhen 麻疹)

Measles is a disease caused by an epidemic virus, manifested by fever, cough, runny nose, conjunctivitis, Koplik's spots, and blotchy red rash. It is also named Ma Zi because the rash has the same size as sesame seeds (Zhi Ma in Chinese). *Xiao Er Yue Zheng Zhi Jue* (Key to Differentiation and Treatment of Disease of Children) 1114 states: "if a patient has reddish complexion, puffy and swollen eye lips, yawning, chills and fever, cough, sneezing, cold extremities, fright and palpitation during sleep, sleepiness, accompanied with rashes, it is an epidemic disease. " It describes the manifestations and epidemic of measles. *You Ke Da Quan* (Encyclopedia of Children) by Zhu Danxi points out the pathology of measles is "toxin in spleen and heat flowering into heart. The most damaged of the zang and fu organ is the lung." *Yi Zong Jing Jie* (Golden Mirror of the Medical Tradition·Teachings on Pox) 1742 suggests "The treatment for measles is first to expel exterior and promote measles." Measles is transmitted by direct contact with infectious droplets, or less commonly, by airborne spread. The only natural hosts of the measles virus are humans. Measles occurs throughout the world, usually in young children, especially from 6 month old to 5 years old. All persons who have not had the disease, or have not been successfully immunized, are susceptible. The incidence of measles is much less after the vaccination has been used in the world, but in recent years, clinically atypical measles has increased. Measles of either type usually clears up on its own in seven to 10 days. Once a person has had a case of the measles, they are almost always immune for life. Complications are rare but may be serious. It was one of the four most critical diseases in ancient times. This is the reason why vaccination is so universally recommended.

Etiology and Pathology

It is due invading measles virus, which invades the lung and stomach/spleen through the mouth and nose, causing accumulation of heat in lungs and stomach. The pathogen is then expelled out through the skin. If the pathogen transforms internally and is not released externally, it causes reverse syndromes of measles.

Pathogen invading the lung and stomach and spleen It is favorable if the pathogen passes out through the skin following the development of measles.

Pathogen invading the lung and Wei The measles toxin invades the lungs and Wei at the beginning stage, causing the exterior Wei to be disordered, and the lung Qi stagnated. The manifestations of exterior Wei syndrome, fever, runny nose and cough are present. It is the early stage.

Excessive heat accumulating in the lungs and stomach If the measles toxin transforms to the spleen and stomach from the exterior of the lungs and Wei, the heat accumulates in the lungs and stomach. This leads to the syndrome of excessive heat in the lung and stomach, which manifests as high fever and thirst. The toxin passes out through the skin and muscles, causing rashes all over the skin. If the rashes go to the extremities, it means that all the toxin has been released from the body. It is the rash stage.

Damage to the lungs and stomach Yin At this stage, fever and rashes are no longer present, with the heat and toxin absent from the skin, however since measles toxin is a Yang pathogen, it tends to damage yin, with the yin injured, it takes time to recover. This is the recovery stage.

Measles toxin involving the interior Severe excessive measles toxin, weak energy of the patient, or incorrect treatment for the illness, may disturb the process of the toxin going outward. When the measles toxin goes inward abnormally, the reversal syndrome occurs.

Measles toxin closing the lungs The excessive toxin abnormally goes inward and closes the lung interiorly. The excessive heat burns the body fluids leading to phlegm, which stagnates and closes the lung qi. Therefore, the syndrome of measles toxin closing the lungs occurs.

Measles toxin attacking the throat The throat is the gate of the lungs and stomach. If excessive toxin goes to the throat along the meridian and blocks the airway, the syndrome of measles attacking throat occurs.

Measles toxin involving the liver and heart

This is due to vital qi being too weak to defend the excessive pathogen. It involves the Jueyin inwardly and abnormally. As a result, the heart orifice is closed, and wind is stirred and flared upward. The syndrome of toxin involving the liver and heart occurs.

In summary, the excessive heat in the lungs and stomach is the main pathology. The syndrome of measles toxin closing the lungs is the most common reversal syndrome.

Diagnosis

Diagnostic Guidelines

Occurs in susceptible children in the winter and spring, in areas where there is an outbreak of, and in children who have a recent history of exposure to measles..

Diagnostic Notes

- Pay attention to inquiring about the epidemiological history and vaccination history.
- Observe the eyes' manifestations and Koplik's spots at the first fever stage.
- Observe the relationship between fever and rash, as well as the rash characteristics.
- Observe the recovery of skin desquamation and pigmentation at the recovery stage.

Pattern Differentiation

Manifestations

Typical manifestations of measles in the clinic are divided into three stages. The first fever stage, starts with a fever that may reach up to 104 °F(40 °C) accompanied by cough, running nose, cold head, conjunctivitis (red eyes) and rashes. Koplik's spots seen inside the mouth are diagnostic for the early stage of measles. In second stage-the rash stage, measles rash is classically described as a generalized, maculopapular, erythematous rash that begins 3~4 days after the fever starts. It starts on the back of the ears and, after a few hours, spreads to the head and neck before spreading to cover most of the body. The rash changes color from red to dark brown after rashes appear in for 2~3 days. In third stage-the recovery stage, symptoms improve and rashes subside according to the order of their rashes appearance. There are small rash scales and pigmentation after the rashes subsides.

Exams and tests

Blood tests may show low WBC, and an increase in lymphocytes. The patient may be checked for measles for serology and in some cases a viral culture may be obtained.

Differentiation of Diagnosis

Common cold and flu

Patients do not have puffy and reddish eye lids, no aversion to light and tears, no Koplik's spots.

Rubella, exantherna subitum, and scarlet fever

It is based on the relationship between initial symptoms, fever and rash, rash characteristics, special signs and recovery of skin manifestations to differentiate them. See the section scarlet on rash where the four rows of diseases are listed in an identification table.

Guidelines of differentiation

Favorable and reverse syndromes should be differentiated first. If manifestations of measles orderly follow the three stages- The first fever stage, the rash stage and the recovery stage, it is a favorable syndrome. If there are symptoms of measles toxin closing the lung, measles toxin attacking the throat, and measles toxin involving liver and heart, it is the reversal syndrome.

Therapeutic Principle

There were doctrines about measles in ancient books, such as "measles is caused by Yang toxin", "measles tends to be cleared with the cool" and "there is no limitation of promoting measles out". It points that promoting measles rash out with clearing and cooling." The therapy is promoting and dispersing for the first fever stage, clearing and detoxicating for the rash stage and nourishing yin for the recovery stage. Clearing heat and toxin is for reverse syndrome, adding opening the lungs and eliminating phlegm for measles toxin closing the lungs, soothing the throat and reducing swelling for measles toxin attacking throat, sedating wind and opening the orifice for toxin involving the heart and liver.

Patterns and treatment

Favorable Syndromes

Toxin invading the lung

Manifestations

Fever with slight chills, stuffy nose with running discharge, sneeze, cough, conjunctive and puffy eye lips, photophobia, tears, fatigue and poor appetite. There are Koplik spots (Koplik spots is ulcerated mucosal lesions marked by necrosis, neutrophilic exudate, and neovascularization. They are described as appearing like "grains of salt on a wet background" and often fade as the maculopapular rash develops. It will gradually disappear after rashes occur), red tongue with thin and yellow coating, floating and purple index finger vein, or floating and rapid pulse.

Treatment Principle Expel exterior pathogen and bring rashes out.

Formula

Xuan Du Fa Biao Tang (Detoxicate and Expel Exterior Decoction) or Yin Qiao San (Honeysuckle and Forsythia Powder).

In the first formula, Sheng Ma (Rhizoma Cimicifugae), Ge Gen (Radix Puerariae) and Fu Ping (Herba Spirodelae) bring the measles rashes out with acrid and cool herbs. Jing Jie (Herbs Seu Flos Schizonepetae Tenuifoliae), Fang Feng (Redix Ledebouriella Divaricatae) and Bo He (Herba Menthae Haplocalycis) assist in promoting the rashes. Jin Yin Hua (Flos Lonicerae Japonicae) and Huang Lian (Rhizoma Coptidis) clear heat and toxin. Qian Hu (Radix Peucedani), Niu Bang Zi (Fructus Arctii), Jie Geng (Radix Platycodi Grandiflori) and Gan Cao (Radix Glycyrrhizae Uralensis) disperse the lungs, eliminate phlegm and soothe the throat. If there is a high fever, add Da Qing Ye (Folium Daqingye) and Pu Gong Ying (Herba Taraxaci Mongolici Cum). If there is severe cough with phlegm, also add Xing Ren (Semen Pruni Armeniacae) and Zhe Bei Mu (Fritillaria Thunbergii).

Excessive heat accumulating in the lungs and stomach

Manifestations

Continuous fever that comes in waves with slight sweating, rashes that appear when the body temperature is higher, anxiety, thirst, conjunctive eyes with tears. The rashes starts behind the ear, then spreads to the head, face, back, chest and four limbs. At the beginning, the thorny rashes are sparse and reddish, but become dense and purple gradually. The tongue is red with a yellow coating, rapid pulse, or there is purple and stagnated index finger vein.

Treatment Principle Clear heat and toxin, promote rashes.

Formula

Qing Jie Tou Biao Tang (Clear, Detoxification and Promote Exterior Decoction.)

In the formula, Ju Hua (Flos Chrysanthemi Morifolii), Sang Ye (Folium Mori Albae), Niu Bang Zi (Fructus Arctii Lappae) and Chan Tui (Periostracum Cicadae) expel wind and clear heat. Jin Yin Hua (Flos Lonicerae Japonicae), Lian Qiao (Fructus Forsythiae Suspensae) and Ban Lan Gen (Radix Isatidis Seu Baphicacanthi) clear heat and detoxifies. If there is high fever, add Bai Hu Tang (White Tiger Decoction). If there are very dense and purple rashes, also add Sheng Di Huang (Radix Rehmanniae Glutinosae) and Mu Dan Pi (Cortex Moutan Radicis). If there is severe cough, add Sang Bai Pi (Cortex Mori Albae Radicis) and Xing Ren (Bitter Apricot Kernel).

Damage to lung and stomach yin

Manifestations

Fever and rashes fade gradually according to the order that the rashes appear, appetite and spirit are better. There are small rash scales and pigmentation after rashes disappear, thirst, red tongue with less coating, thin and rapid pulse.

Treatment Principle Nourish the yin of lungs and stomach, clear the lingering pathogen

Formula

Sha Shen Mai Dong Tang (Glehnia and Ophiopogonis Decoction)

In the formula, Sha Shen (Radix Adenophorae Seu Glehniae), Mai Men Dong (Tuber Ophiopogonis Japonici), Tian Hua Fen (Radix Trichosanthes), Yu Zhu (Rhizoma Polygonti Odorati) and Sang Ye (Folium Mori Albae) nourish Yin and clear heat of the lungs and stomach. Bai Bian Dou (Dolichos Lablab) and Gan Cao (Radix Glycyrrhizae Uralensis) strengthen the spleen and stomach. If there is lower grade fever, add Di Gu Pi (Cortex Lycii Radicis) and Zhi Mu (Rhizome Anemarrhenae). If there is cough, add Xing Ren (Bitter Apricot Kernel) and Pi Pa Ye(Eriobotryae Japobicae). If there is constipation, add Gua Lou Ren (Semen Trichosanthis) and Huo Ma Ren (Hemp Seed).

Reverse Syndromes

Measles toxin closing the lungs

Manifestations

High fever not fading, cough and shortness of breath, nasal flaring, purple complexion and cyanosis of the lips, concentrated skin rashes, restlessness, red tongue with yellow coating, rapid pulse, or purple stagnated index finger vein.

Treatment Principle Clear heat and toxin, unlock the lung and eliminate phlegm.

Formula

Ma Xing Shi Gan Tang (Ephedra, Apricot, Licorice and Gypsum Decoction)

In the formula, Ma Huang (Ephedra) and Shi Gao (Gypsum) clear heat of the lungs and stomach. Xing Ren (Bitter Apricot Kernel) assists Ma Huang to relieve asthma and stops cough, and accompanying Gan Cao (Radix Glycyrrhizae Uralensis) resolves phlegm and stops cough. If there is high fever without fading, add Huang Qin (Radix Scutellariae Baicalensis), Lian Qiao (Fructus Forsythiae Suspensae) and Yu Xing Cao (Houttuynia Cordata). If there is severe shortness of breath with a lot phlegm, also add Ting Li Zi (Lepidium Apetalum), Zhu Li (Succus Bambusae) and Gua Lou (Fructus Trichosanthis). If there is abdominal distention, add Da Huang (Radix et Rhizoma Rhei) and Mang Xiao (Mirabilite). If there are purple lips and complexion, add Hong Hua (Flos Carthami Tinctorii) and Dan Shen (Radix Salviae Miltiorrhizae). If there are rashes that are difficult to clear, add Ge Gen (Radix Puerariae) and Sheng Ma (Rhizoma Cimicifugae).

Measles toxin attacking the throat

Manifestations

High fever not fading, sore throat, reddish and swollen throat, cough with a lot of phlegm, anxiety and restlessness, purple complexion and cyanosis of the lips, concentrated skin rashes, red tongue with yellow coating, rapid pulse, or purple stagnated index vein.

Treatment Principle Clear heat and toxin, soothe the throat and reduce swelling

Formula: Niu Bang Gan Jie Tang (Lappae, Licorice and Grandiflori Decoction)

In the formula, She Gan (Belamcanda Chinesis), Xuan Shen (Radix Scrophulariae Ningpoensis), Jie Geng (Radix Platycodi Grandiflori), Niu Bang Zi (Fructus Arctii) and Gan Cao (Radix Glycyrrhizae Uralensis) clear heat and toxin, disperse the lung and soothe the throat. Huang Qin (Scutellaria Baicalensis), Jin Yin Hua (Flos Lonicerae Japonicae), Lian Qiao (Fructus Forsythiae Suspensae), Zhi Zi (Fructus Gardeniae Jasminoidis) clear heat and purge fire, and Gua Lou (Fructus Trichosanthis) and Zhe Bei Mu (Fritillaria Thunbergii) eliminate phlegm and resolve masses. If there is constipation, add Da Huang (Radix et Rhizoma Rhei) and Mang Xiao (Mirabilite). If there is shortness of breath, purple complexion and lips, refer the patient to MD or ER.

Toxin involving the liver and heart

Manifestations

High fever not fading, restlessness, delirium, concentrated skin rashes, crimson tongue with yellow coating, rapid pulse, or purple stagnated index finger vein.

Treatment Principle Clear heat and cool the Ying, sedate wind and open orifice.

Formula

Qing Ying Tang (Clear the Nutritive Level Decoction) and Ling Yang Gou Teng Tang (Antelope Horn and Uncaria Decoction).

In the formula, Shui Niu Jiao (Cornu Bubali), Sheng Di Huang (Radix Rehmanniae Glutinosae), Mu Dan Pi (Cortex Moutan Radicis), Xuan Shen (Radix Ccrophulariae Ningpoensis), Ling Yang Jiao (Antilope Horn), Gou Teng (Ramulus Cum Uncis Uncariae) and Ju Hua (FlosCchrysanthemi Morifolii) clear heat, cool the liver and sedate wind. Bai shao (Radix Paeoniae Lactiflorae) and Gan Cao (Radix Glycyrrhizae Uralensis) soften the liver and relax spasm. Shi Chang Pu (Rhizoma Acori Graminei) and Yu Jin (Tuber Curcumae) eliminate phlegm, open orifice and wake up the spirit. Zi Cao (Radix Arnebiae Seu Lithospermi) cools the blood, clears heat and promotes rashes. If there is high fever, coma and convulsion, add Zi Xue Dan (Purple Snow Special Pill), or An Gong Niu Huang Wan (Calm the Palace Pill with Cattle Gallstone).

Other Therapy

Patent herbs

- Yin Qiao Jie Du Pian (Honeysuckle and Forsythia Detoxicating Pills), taken orally 3~6 g per time, 2 times per day. It is used for early stage due to excessive heat.
- Hei Chun Dan (Return of Spring Special Pill),taken orally 1~5 pills per time, 1~2 times per day. It is used for measles rash stage.

Topical therapy

Ma Huang (Herba Ephedra), Fu Ping (Herba spirodelae), Yuan Tuo (Eryngium Foetidum) He Xi Liu (Cacumen Tamaricis) 15g of each wrapped together, boil it 250 cc water for about 15 minutes. Put the warm decoction on the face, neck, back, extremities with a towel. This can promote the rashes out.

Prevention and care

Once the child has contracted the disease they should be isolated until the measles rash is gone for 5 days. If there are complicating factors such as pneumonia, they are isolated for 10 days after rash is gone. Children who have had possible contact with the virus or measles patient should be observed for 21 days.

Exanthema Subitum (Nai Ma奶 麻)

Exantherna Subitum is an acute and epidemic disease caused by wind and heat, manifested with sudden fever lasting around 3~4 days, and rashes that occur after the fever fades. Since it is children's disease, generally under two years old, and looks similar to measles, it is named as Nai Ma (baby measles). The causes, location and therapy of exantherna subitun were mentioned in On the Measles and Pox (1713), it said "Exantherna subitum and hives are caused by wind-heat in the spleen and lungs, treated with the expel exterior decoction of Schizonepeta and Ledebouriella. This formula can strongly expel wind and clear heat." There is no specific vaccine against or treatment in main stream medicine for exanthema subitum. Children can get long term immunity. Most children with the disease are not seriously ill. It often occurs in spring and winter.

Etiology and pathology

Exantherna Subitum is due to wind-heat that invades the lungs and stomach through the mouth and nose, excessive heat accumulating in the lungs and stomach, which is expelled out through the skin.

Pathogen stagnating the lungs and stomach The pathogen invades the lungs and stomach, stagnates long term and turns into heat. Excessive heat accumulates in the lungs and stomach, which results in high fever and reddish throat. The lung Qi fails to disperse, resulting in mild cough and runny nose. There is spleen and stomach disharmony, causing poor appetite, vomiting and diarrhea.

Pathogen letting out through the skin Heat toxin enters the lungs and stomach, there is fighting between Zheng Qi and evil Qi, if the Zheng Qi is stronger than evil, then the evil fades, the pathogen is let out through the skin and the fever goes down.

Manifestations and signs

Typical manifestations in the clinic are divided into two stages.

The fever stage and rash appearing stage At the fever stage, the disease typically begins with a sudden high fever (102.2~104 °F). This can cause, in rare cases, febrile convulsions due to the sudden rise in body temperature, but in many cases the child appears normal.

The rashes appearing stage After 3~4 days the fever subsides, and just as the child appears to be recovering, a red rash appears. This usually begins on the trunk, spreading to the legs and neck. The rash is not itchy and may last 1 to 2 days. In contrast, a child suffering from measles would usually appear more infirm, with symptoms of conjunctivitis, coryza, cough, and the rash would affect the face and last for several days. Liver dysfunction can occur in rare cases.

Diagnosis

Diagnostic Guidelines

There is a higher occurrence in the winter and spring. It happens in children under the age of two years old. The children have recent history of exposure to Exanthema Subitum

Blood test: It may show blood leukocytes reduced and lymphocytes relatively increased. The blood test may also find antibodies for roseola.

Diagnostic Notes

- Pay attention to the age of patient.
- Observe the spirit and do a thorough physical exam during fever stage.
- Note the relationship between fever and the appearance of rashes.

Differentiation of Diagnosis

Common cold and flu

It is difficult to distinguish the fever stage of exantherna subitum from the fever of common cold and flu. The cough and running nose are more obvious, and rarely have high fever last more than 3~4 days.

Measles, rubella and scarlet fever

The relationship between initial symptoms of fever and rash, the rash characteristics, the presence of special signs, and the recovery of skin manifestations are used to differentiate them.

Therapeutic principle

Focus on clearing heat and toxin. If there is lingering toxin inside, also clear the lingering toxin.

Pattern Differentiation

Guidelines of differentiation

Differentiate between the mild and the severe. If the fever is mild, the child has good spirit, the rash is diffuse and accompanying symptoms are mild, it is a mild syndrome. If there is a high fever, anxiety, or even convulsion, coma, and rashes is more, it is a severe syndrome.

Patterns and treatment

Pathogen stagnating in the lung and stomach

Manifestations

Sudden high fever that does not abate, mild red throat, mild cough, runny nose, poor appetite, normal spirit, red tongue with thin white or thin yellow coating, floating and rapid pulse, or floating and purple index finger vein.

Treatment Principle Clear heat and toxin

Formula

Yin Qiao San (Honeysuckle and Forsythia Powder) and Bai Hu Tang (White Tiger Decoction).

In the formula, Jing Jie(Herbs Seu Flos Schizonepetae Tenuifoliae), Bo He (Herba Menthae Haplocalycis), Dan Dou Chi (Semen Sojae Praeparatum) expel wind and release exterior. Niu Bang Zi (Fructus Arctii), Jie Geng (Radix Platycodi Grandiflori) and Gan Cao (Radix Glycyrrhizae Uralensis) disperse the lung and soothe the throat. Jin yin Hua (Flos Lonicerae Japonicae) and Lian Qiao (Rhizoma Coptidis) clear heat and toxin. Shi Gao (Gypsum), Zhi Mu (Rhizome Anemarrhenae) and Lu Gen (Rhizoma Phragmitis Communis) clear heat and generate fluids. If there are convulsions, add Chan Tui (Periostracum Cicadae) and Gou Teng (Ramulus Cum Uncis Uncariae).

Pathogen expelled through the skin

Manifestations

Fever that suddenly subsides, a red and slight purple rash on the trunk and hips, but mild on the extremities. It may last 1 to 2 days. Red tongue with thin yellow coating, thin and rapid pulse.

Treatment Principle Clear heat and toxin, cool the blood

Formula: Qing Re Liang Xue Tang (Clear Heat and Cool Blood Decoction).

In the formula, Dan Zhu Ye (Herba Loptatheri Gracilis), Lian Qiao (Rhizoma Coptidis) and Zi Hua Di Ding (Herba Cum Radice Violae Yedoensitis) clear lingering heat and toxin. Sheng Di Huang (Radix Rehmanniae Glutinosae), Mu Dan Pi (Cortex Moutan Radicis)2~4g and Chi Shao (Radix Paeoniae Rubra) cools blood.

If the fever subsides without the other symptoms and the child's spirit is good, the nursing to recovery and prevention should be the focus.

Other Therapy

Patents

- Yin Huang Kou Fu Ye (Honeysuckle and Scutellariae Liquid) taken orally 5~10cc for per time, 3 times per day. It is used for pathogen accumulating in the lungs and stomach.

Acupuncture

Du14, LI 11, LI4 and ST36. Reducing manipulation 2~3 minutes, take the needles out. 1~2 times per day. It is used for high fever.

Topical Therapy

Sang Ye (Folium Mori Albae)15g, Lian Qiao (Fructus Forsythiae Suspensae)10g, Ban Lan Gen (Radix Isatidis Seu Baphicacanthi)15g, Chan Tui (Periostracum Cicadae)10g. Decoct all of the herbs 20 minutes, then remove the herbs. The child takes a bath with the herbal decoction. Do this for 2~3 days. It is used for pathogens accumulating in the lungs and stomach.

Prevention and care

- Isolate the child for about 10 days.

- Try not to let infants and young children go to public places in the winter and spring.
- High fever in children should be treated promptly to prevent convulsion.

Rubella (Feng Sha风 痧)

Rubella is an acute and epidemic disease caused by wind and heat, manifested with mild fever, cough, runny nose, pink rashes and swollen glands or lymph nodes behind the ears and neck. Typically rubella is transmitted via airborne droplet emission from the upper respiratory tract of active cases (it can be passed along through the breath of an infected person). The disease has an incubation period of 2 to 3 weeks. In most people the disease is rapidly eliminated. These children are a significant source of infection to other children and, more importantly, to pregnant female contacts. It mostly affects children in the 5-9 year old age group, but may also occur in adults. Since the introduction of the rubella vaccine, occurrences have become rare in those countries. Rubella infection of children and adults is usually mild, self-limiting and often asymptomatic. Rubella in a pregnant woman can cause congenital rubella syndrome, with potentially devastating consequences for the developing fetus. Children who are infected with rubella before birth are at risk for growth retardation; mental retardation; malformations of the heart and eyes; deafness; and liver, spleen, and bone marrow problems.

Etiology and pathology

Rubella is due to wind heat that invades the lungs and Wei Qi, and is expelled out through the skin. Occasionally, the excessive pathogen may invade the interior.

Pathogen stagnating the lungs and Wei Qi The pathogen invades the lungs and defensive Qi, which leads to disharmony between the lungs and Wei (defensive) Qi, resulting in mild fever, cough and runny nose. The pathogen expelled out from the skin, shows as a slight red rashes on the skin.

Flaming of heat in the Qi and Ying If the pathogen is particularly strong, it transfers into the Qi and Ying level; high fever, delirium, and convulsion occurs. It also may cause symptoms in other organ and cause additional systems.

Diagnosis

Diagnostic guidelines

This mostly occurs in the winter and spring. It happens between 5 and 9 years old. The children have recent history of exposure to Rubella.

Manifestations and signs

Typical manifestations in the clinic are divided into two stages. The before-rash stage and the rash appearing stage. The before-rash stage presents with swollen glands or lymph nodes behind the ears and neck for ½ ~1 day, the symptoms are mild, such as mild fever, cough, sore throat, runny nose. During the rash-appearing stage rashes occur after fever 1~2 days, the rashes are pink with itching, and rashes disappear 2~3 days after appearing, with no desquamation and no pigmentation. Blood test may show a reduction in blood leukocytes with lymphocytes relatively increased. Rubella virus specific IgM antibodies are present in people recently infected by Rubella virus but these antibodies can persist for over a year and a positive test result needs to be interpreted with caution. The presence of these antibodies along with, the characteristic rash, or the development of the rash shortly thereafter, confirms the diagnosis.

Diagnostic Notes

- Pay attention the age of the patient.
- Observe the relationship between the fever and the appearance of rashes.
- Check the lymph nodes behind the ears and neck.

Differentiation of Diagnosis

Rubella needs to be distinguished from measles, exantherna subitum and scarlet fever.

It is based on the relationship between initial symptoms of fever and rash, rash characteristics, special signs, and the recovery of skin manifestations to differentiate them.

Therapeutic principle

Focus on expelling wind and clearing heat and toxin for pathogen stagnating in the lungs and defensive Qi. It also may clear heat and toxin, cool blood for flaming of heat at Qi and Ying levels.

Pattern Differentiation

Guidelines of differentiation

Differentiate between the mild and the severe. If the fever is mild, the child patient has good spirit, diffuse rash and accompanying symptoms are mild, it is mild syndrome due to pathogen stagnating in the lungs and Wei level. If there is a high fever, anxiety, dense and purple rashes, or even convulsions and coma, it is severe syndrome due to heat flaming in the Qi and Ying levels.

Patterns and treatment

Pathogen stagnating the lungs and defensive Qi

Manifestations

Mild fever, cough, runny nose, diffuse and pink rashes with itching, swollen lymph nodes behind the ears and neck, red tongue with thin yellow coating, floating and rapid pulse.

Treatment Principle Expel wind, clear heat and toxin.

Formula

Yin Qiao San (Honeysuckle and Forsythia Powder).

In the formula, Jing Jie (Herbs Seu Flos Schizonepetae Tenuifoliae), Bo He (Herba Menthae Haplocalycis), Dan Dou Chi (Semen Sojae Praeparatum) expel wind-heat. Jin Yin Hua (Flos LoniceraeJjaponicae) and Lian Qiao (Rhizoma Coptidis) clear heat and toxin. Niu Bang Zi (Fructus Arctii), Jie Geng (Radix Platycodi Grandiflori) and Gan Cao (Radix Glycyrrhizae Uralensis) disperse the lung and soothe throat. Lu Gen (Rhizoma Phragmitis Communis) clear heat and generate fluids. If there are swollen lymph nodes, add. Xia Ku Cao (Spica Prunella Vulgaris) and Pu Gong Ying (Herba Taraxaci Mongolici Cum) clear heat and toxins, and resolve nodules. If there is skin itching, add Chan Tui (Periostracum Cicadae) and Bai Ji Li (Fructus Tribuli Terrestris) to expel wind and stop itching.

Flaming of heat in the Qi and Ying

Manifestations

High fever, thirst, dense and purple rashes, severe itching, swollen and painful lymph nodes behind the ears, red tongue with yellow coating, full and rapid pulse.

Treatment Principle Clear heat and cool blood.

Formula

Tou Zhen LiangJie Tang (Expel Rashes and Cool Decoction).

In the formula, Sang Ye (Folium Mori Albae), Niu Bang Zi (Fructus Arctii Lappae) and Chan Tui (Periostracum Cicadae) expel wind and clear heat. Jin Yin Hua (Flos Lonicerae Japonicae), Lian Qiao (Fructus Forsythiae Suspensae), Huang Qin (Radix Scutellariae Baicalensis) and Zi Hua Di Ding (Herba Cum Radice Violae Yedoensitis) clear heat and toxin. Chi Shao (Radix Paeoniae Rubra) and Hong Hua (Flos Carthami Tinctorii) cools and invigorate blood. If there is severe thirst, also add Shi Hu (Dendrobium Stem) and Lu Gen (Rhizoma Phragmitis Communis) to clear heat and generate fluid. If there is constipation, add Da Huang (Radix et Rhizoma Rhei) and Mang Xiao (Mirabilite) to encourage bowel movement and clear heat. If the syndrome is severe, use Qing Wen Bai Du Yin (Clear Epidemics and Overcome Toxin Decoction).

Other Therapy

Patent herbs

- Ban Lan Gen Chong Ji (Radix Isatidis Seu Baphicacanthi Granule) oral taking 0.5~1bag per time, 3 times per day. It is used for pathogen stagnating in the lung and Wei.
- San Huang Pian (Three Yellow Pills) taken orally 1~2 pills per time, three times per day. It is used for flaming of heat in the Qi and Ying level.

Topical Therapy

Heat the Hua Sheng You (Peanut Oil) 50g. After it cools a little, add Bo He (Herba Menthae Haplocalycis) 30g. Remove the herbs after it cools down. Smear the oil on the local skin. It is used to stop itching.

Prevention and care

- Isolate patients for days after the rashes subside.
- During the epidemic season, keep susceptible children and pregnant women away from public places. During early pregnancy exposure should be minimized to avoid infection.
- Susceptible children, premarital woman should do rubella vaccine.
- The patients must pay attention to rest, adequate water supply, and should eat foods that are easily digestible and nutritious.
- Avoid scratching the skin in order to prevent skin infections.

Scarlet Fever (Dan Sha 丹痧)

Scarlet fever is an acute and epidemic disease caused by a warm febrile and toxin, manifested by fever, sore throat or with pus on the tonsil, cough, runny nose, scarlet macules and rashes on the whole body. It is also named as Lan Hou Dan Sha (Rotten throat and scarlet fever) since it causes throat abscesses). It was described in the Qing dynasty (1746), Lin Zheng Zhi Nan Yi An (A guide to clinical cases and practice) which noted "The epidemic pathogen distributes in the three Jiao, spirit and mind through the mouth and the nose with breathing. It is not due to wind cold invading exteriorly and stagnating interiorly. This is why the treatments to expel the exterior and purge stagnation may incorrectly damage fluids. It is quite different from the six meridian differentiation of the Shang Han Lun. The patient has a sore throat, and scarlet rashes, deep red tongue, anxiety and delirium, the cause is epidemic infection attacking the upper Jiao and adversely invading Tan Zhong (Ren17). The treatment is to clear blood vesicles and to prevent the closing syndrome, strongly clear heat and toxin to expel the epidemic." It mentioned the name, manifestations and treatments for the scarlet fever. Scarlet fever is usually spread by the aerosol route (inhalation) but may also be spread by skin contact. It mostly affects children ages 3~15, especially the 3~8 year old age group. Before the availability of antibiotics, scarlet fever was a major cause of death. It also sometimes caused late complications, such as convulsion, edema (glomerulonephritis), Bi syndrome, and palpitation (endocarditis), all of which were protracted and often fatal at the time.

Etiology and pathology

Scarlet fever is due to an epidemic toxin of the warm febrile type, which invades the lungs and stomach through the mouth and nose. The toxin flames upward to the throat and forces the Ying and blood interiorly. The toxin is expelled out through the skin.

Toxin invading the Wei

The throat is the gate of lungs and stomach. The toxin accumulates in the lungs and stomach, it starts in the skin, showing exterior symptoms, such as fever and chills. It quickly moves inside and transforms into fire, showing symptoms of Qi level, such as high fever and thirst. The toxin goes upwards to the throat along the meridians, causing swollen throat sometimes with pus.

Flaming of heat in Qi and Ying Severe toxin in the Qi level causes high fever, thirst, swollen throat with pus. The toxin is pushed to the skin, resulting in deep red rashes. The toxin may involve the Jueyin meridian, and cause delirium convulsion, or other severe syndromes of the Zang Fu organs, such as exhaustion syndrome of the heart and kidney.

Yin vacuity of the lungs and stomach The epidemic toxin of the warm febrile type is yang pathogen and tends to consume yin. The yin and fluids is weakened after the toxin is expelled, resulting in symptoms of yin vacuity of the lung and stomach. If the toxin lingers in the body, it damages heart Qi, resulting in palpitation. If the toxin floods to the joints, it causes swollen and painful joints. If it invades inside and damages the lung, spleen and kidney, it disturbs the water metabolism, resulting in edema.

Diagnosis

Diagnostic Guidelines

This disease occurs more often in the winter and spring. It happens in children between 5 and 9 years old. The children have recent history of exposure to scarlet fever.

Manifestations and signs

Typical manifestations in the clinic are divided into three stages, the before-rash stage, the rash- appearing stage and the recovery stage. In the before-rash stage, the patient has a high fever for 24 hours, swollen and reddish throat which may have pus. In the rashes stage, the patient has rashes that occur 24 hours after the onset of the fever in one day, which generally begins on the chest, armpits and behind the ears. The rash is the most striking sign of scarlet fever. It usually appears first on the neck and face (often leaving a clear, unaffected area around the mouth). It looks like a bad sunburn with tiny bumps, and it may itch. It then spreads to the chest, back, and finally to the rest of the body. In the body creases, especially around the axillae (underarms) and elbows, the rash forms the classic red streaks known as Pastia lines. On very dark skin, the streaks may appear darker than the rest of the skin. Areas of rash usually turn white (or paler brown, with dark complected skin) when pressed on. The tongue shows bright red with a "strawberry" appearance. In the recovery stage, by the fourth day of the disease, the rash begins to fade and peeling begins. This phase begins with flakes peeling from the face. Peeling from the palms and around the fingers occurs about a week later.

Blood test

Complete blood count findings characteristic of scarlet fever would show marked leukocytosis with neutrophilia and increased eosinophils, high erythrocyte sedimentation rate (ESR) and C-reactive protein (CRP) (both indications of inflammation), and elevation of antistreptolysin O titer.

Diagnostic Notes

- -Pay attention to epidemiology currently occurring, as well as season and ages of patients.
- -Check the throat carefully
- Observe the relationship between fever and the appearance of rashes, and the patient's complexion and tongue.
- Observe the peeled skin after the rashes fade.
- Check the following lab exams in time, such as CBC, eosinophils, erythrocyte sedimentation rate (ESR), C-reactive protein (CRP), antistreptolysin O and Blood culture.

Differentiation of Diagnosis

Tonsillitis: It is difficult to distinguish from tonsillitis at the early stage, but scarlet fever will have deep red rashes one day after the fever. Tonsillitis does not manifest with any rashes.

Scarlet fever needs to be distinguished from measles, exanthema subitum and rubella.

Differences Among the Four Warm Febrile Diseases that Have Rashes

Names	Measles	Rubella	Exanthema Subitum	Scarlet Fever
Early symptoms	Fever, cough, running nose, tears, Koplik's spots	Mild fever, cough, running nose, swollen glands or lymph nodes behind the ears and neck.	Sudden high fever, no other symptoms.	high fever, swollen and reddish throat with pus
Fever relates To rashes	After fever 3~4 days, rashes occurs at peak fever	After fever ½~1day, rashes occurs with mild fever.	Rashes occurs at after fever 3~4 days and the fever fades	Rash occurs 24 hours after onset of fever
Character of rashes	Red rash starts on the back of the ears spreads to the head and neck, then cover most of the body. The rash changes color from red to dark brown in 2~3 days. It becomes light, then fades.	Pink rashes with itching occur 1~2 days after onset of fever, it covers the whole body in 1 day. It disappears after 2~3 days, no desquamation and no pigmentation.	Red rash appears, begins on the trunk, spreading to the legs and neck. The rash is not itchy and lasts 1 to 2 days.	bad sunburn rashes with tiny bumps in all body, rash forms the classic red streaks known as Pastia lines.

	Koplik's spots	No	No	Pastia lines, pale-brown lips, strawberry tongue
Special Sign				
Recovery stage	small, peeled with pigmentation	No peeling and no pigmentation	No peeling and no pigmentation	flaking and peeling without pigmentation

Pattern Differentiation

Guidelines of differentiation

Differentiate between the mild and severe syndrome. If the fever is low, tonsils are mildly swollen with little pus, good spirit, diffuse rashes and the other accompanied symptoms are mild, it is a mild syndrome. On the other hand, if there is high fever, anxiety, swollen tonsils with pus, dense and purple rashes or even convulsions, and coma, it is severe syndrome.

Treatment principle

The main principle is to clear heat and toxin, cool blood and soothe the throat. Clear heat and expel exterior, soothe the throat while the pathogen is in the Wei and Qi level. Clear Qi and cool the Ying, clear heat toxin, and soothe the throat for the middle stage of flaming of the Qi and Ying levels. Nourish Yin and clear heat, generate fluid and moisten throat after the rashes fade.

Patterns and treatment

Pathogen stagnating the lungs and defensive level

Manifestations: sudden fever and chills, headache, thirst, swollen tonsils possibly with pus, flushed of the skin, undistinguished rashes, red tongue with prickles, thin and yellow tongue coating. Floating and rapid pulse, or floating and purple index vein.

259

Treatment Principle Expel exterior and clear heat, soothe the throat and promote rashes.

Formula

Jie Ji Tou Sha Tang(Relax Muscles and Promote Rash Decoction)

In the formula, Jing Jie (Herbs Seu Flos Schizonepetae Tenuifoliae), Fu Ping (Herba Spirodelae), Chan Tui (Periostracum Cicadae) and Ge Gen (Radix Puerariae) clear heat and bring the measles rashes out. Jin yin Hua (Flos Lonicerae Japonicae) and Lian Qiao (Rhizoma Coptidis) clear heat toxin and bring pathogens out. Shi Gao (Gypsum), Ban Lan Gen (Radix Isatidis Seu Baphicacanthi) and Pu Gong Ying (Herba Taraxaci Mongolici Cum) clear heat and purge fire toxin. Niu Bang Zi (Fructus Arctii), Jie Geng (Radix Platycodi Grandiflori), She Gan (Belamcanda Chinesis) and Gan Cao (Radix Glycyrrhizae Uralensis) clear heat and soothe the throat. If there is an obviously swollen throat with pus, also add Wu Wei Xiao Du yin (Five Ingredients Clear Toxin Decoction). Yin Qiao San (Honeysuckle and Forsythia Powder) and Bai Hu Tang (White Tiger Decoction) modified also are used for this syndrome.

Flaming heat in the Qi and Ying

Manifestations

Persistent high fever, anxiety, thirst, flushed complexion, pale and purple lips, swollen tonsils with pus, dense and purple reddish rashes, strawberry tongue, full and rapid pulse.

Treatment Principle Clear Qi and cool Ying, release toxin and soothe the throat.

Formula

Liang Ying Qing Qi Tang(Cool Ying and Clear Qi Decoction).

In the formula, Jin Yin Hua (Flos Lonicerae Japonicae), Lian Qiao (Rhizoma Coptidis), Shi Gao (Gypsum), Huang Qin (Radix

Scutellariae Baicalensis), Zhi Zi (Fructus Gardeniae Jasminoidis) and Dan Zhu Ye (Herba Loptatheri Gracilis) clear heat toxin of the qi level. Shui Niu Jiao (Cornu Bubali), Sheng Di Huang (Radix Rehmanniae Glutinosae), Mu Dan Pi (Cortex Moutan Radicis) and Chi Shao (Radix Paeoniae Rubra) cool the Ying level, release toxin and activate blood. Xuan Shen (Radix Scrophulariae Ningpoensis), Ban Lan Gen (Radix Isatidis Seu Baphicacanthi) and She Gan (Belamcanda Chinesis) resolve toxin and soothe the throat. Sheng Di Huang (Radix Rehmanniae Glutinosae), Shi Hu (Dendrobium Stem) and Shi Hu (Dendrobium Stem) clear heat, generate fluids and nourish Yin. If there are rashes on the skin but they can't fully express, also add Ge Gen (Radix Puerariae) and Fu Ping (Herba Spirodelae) help the measles rashes express. Qing Wen Bai Du Yin (Clear Epidemics and Overcome Toxin Decoction) is also used for this syndrome.

Yin vacuity of the lungs and stomach

Manifestations

The fever and swollen tonsils gradually fade, the rashes gradually disappear, but the patient has peeled skin, dry cough, dry lips, poor appetite, red tongue with peeled coating, thin and rapid pulse.

Treatment Principle Nourish yin and clear heat, generate fluid and moisten the throat.

Formula

Sha Shen Mai Dong Tang (Glehnia and Ophiopogonis Decoction)
   In the formula, Sha Shen (Radix Adenophorae Seu Glehniae), Mai Men Dong (Tuber Ophiopogonis Japonici), Tian Hua Fen (Radix Trichosanthes), Yu Zhu (Rhizoma Polygonti Odorati) and Sang Ye (Folium Mori Albae) nourish yin and clear heat of the lungs and stomach. Bai Bian Dou (Dolichos Lablab) and Gan Cao (Radix Glycyrrhizae Uralensis) strengthen the spleen and stomach. If there is lower grade fever, add Di Gu Pi (Cortex Lycii Radicis) and Yin Chai Hu (Stelaria Dihotoma). If there is poor appetite,

add Sheng Mai Ya (Fresh Fructus Hordei Vulgaris Germinantus) and Sheng Gu Ya (Fresh Fructus Oryzae Sativae Germinantus). If there is constipation, add Huo Ma Ren (Hemp Seed) and Zhi Mu (Rhizome Anemarrhenae).

If the patient has complications, such as palpitations, Bi syndrome or edema, refer to the related chapters.

Other Therapy

Patent herbs

- Liang Ge San (Cool Diaphragm Powder) taken orally 3~6g per time, 2 times per day. It is used for pathogen stagnating in the lung and Wei with constipation.
- Shuang Huang Liang Kou Fu Ye(Double Coptis Liquid) Oral taking 5~10ml per time, 3 times per day. It is used for flaming of heat in the Qi and Ying levels.

Topical therapy

Bing Peng san (Borneolum and Borax Powder) is blown at the tonsil. 2~3 times per day. It is used for swollen tonsils with pus.

If antibiotics are used for Scarlet Fever, it can shorten the course of treatment and reduce complications. It is necessary to refer the patient to visit an MD.

Prevention and care

- Isolate patients for 7 days.
- During the epidemic season, keep them away from public places.
- Susceptible children and premarital woman should get the rubella vaccination.
- The patients should get adequate rest, water, and should eat foods that are easily digestible and nutritious.
- Check the heart and urine in one month, make sure there are no complications.

Chickenpox (Shui Dou水痘)

Chickenpox is an epidemic disease caused by a warm febrile pathogen, manifested by fever, rashes and blisters on the skin with itching. The fluid of the blisters is clear and watery, the blisters look like oval-shaped beans, it is also named as Shui Dou (Water Bean). *Xiao Er Wei Sheng Zhong Wei Fan Lun* (General Hygiene of Pediatrics) 1156 notes"it is named as chickenpox since the blister's skin is very thin, and easily broken and dried". It pointed out the disease name and characters of the blisters. *Yi Zong Jing Jie* (Golden Mirror of the Medical Tradition Teachings on Pox) 1742 notes "Chickenpox is caused by damp-heat; some of the symptoms are similar to those of smallpox, but the blister of chickenpox has clear water inside of it that is easily dried and no pus. The main remedies are Jing Fang Bai Du San (Schizonepeta and Ledebouriella Antiphlogistic Powder) and modified Dao Chi San (Guide Out the Red Powder)." The book points out the cause, characteristics and therapy of chickenpox. The disease is most commonly observed in children, particularly under 10 years old. It is an airborne disease which spreads easily through coughing or sneezing by ill individuals or through direct contact with secretions from the rash. It occurs year-round, more common in the winter and spring. It is highly contagious, it easily spreads in collective institutions of children. The prognosis of chickenpox is generally good and the complications are rare. The blisters do not leave scars. However, in the patient who has immunodeficiency, have taken or is taking corticosteroids or immunosuppressive therapy, who is suffering from malignant diseases, or suffering from the severe case of chicken pox, it may injure internal organs and can even become life-threatening.

Etiology and pathology

Chickenpox is due to an epidemic toxin, which invades the lungs and stomach (spleen) through the mouth and nose with internal dampness. The toxin is leaked out to the skin.

263

Pathogen stagnating the lungs and Wei level The pathogen invades the lungs and defensive Qi, which leads to disharmony between the lungs and Wei(defensive), resulting in fever, cough and runny nose. The pathogen stagnates spleen and stomach with internal dampness leaks to the skin.

Patterns

Flaming heat at Qi and Ying levels If the pathogen is overly excessive, it transfers into the Qi and Ying levels, resulting in high fever, anxiety and thirst. The heat toxin with dampness leaks into the skin, causing severe blisters. If the pathogen invades the heart and liver, it results in convulsion and coma. It also may affect other organs' symptoms.

Diagnosis

Diagnostic guidelines

This disease occurs more often in the winter and spring. The disease spreads in the same area. The children have a recent history of exposure to chickenpox.

Manifestations and signs

The skin manifestations are rash and macules, which blisters that fade and in patches. It begins as red rash and macules, and quickly becomes herpes and blisters that are oval-shaped. They are large and small mixed, mainly located in the trunk, but also on the head, face, mouth, throat, conjunctiva, and genital mucosa. It may be accompanied by fever, cough, and runny nose. Blood test may show blood leukocytes reduced and lymphocytes that are relatively increased. Confirmation of the diagnosis can be sought through either examination of the fluid within the vesicles of the rash, or by testing the blood for evidence of an acute immunologic response.

Diagnostic Notes

- Inquire about the history of previous epidemic infections.
- Observe the relationship between fever and the appearance of rashes.
- Test blood for evidence of an acute immunologic response, if it doesn't have typical manifestations.

Differentiation of Diagnosis

Impetigo It is a highly contagious bacterial skin infection most common among pre-school children. It often occurs in summer, begins as a red sore which soon breaks, leaking pus or thick fluid, and forms a honey-colored scab, followed by a red mark. Sores are not painful, but may be itchy. Touching or scratching the sores may easily spread the infection to other parts of the body.

Papular urticaria It is frequently caused by allergic reactions. It looks like small, raised patches of skin that turn into firm, reddish-brown bumps at the site of old insect bites. Bumps are usually very itchy, and are typically found in clusters on exposed areas such as the face, neck, arms, and legs.

Therapeutic principle

The main principle is to clear heat and toxin, eliminate dampness. Expel wind, clear heat and toxin, eliminate dampness for pathogen stagnating the lungs and Wei. Clear Qi and cool the Ying, clear heat toxin and eliminate dampness for flaming heat of the Qi and Ying.

Pattern Differentiation

Guide lines of differentiation

Differentiate between the mild and severe. If the fever is mild, rashes are loosely distributed, the fluid in the rashes is clear, it is the mild syndrome. If there is high fever, anxiety, dense and purple rashes, the fluid inside is thick, it is the severe syndrome.

Pathogen stagnating in the lungs and stomach

Manifestations: mild fever, cough, sneezing and running nose, loose rashes, light-red rashes, fluid in the rashes is clear, red tongue with thin white or thin yellow and greasy coating, floating and rapid pulse, or floating and purple index vein.

Treatment Principle Clear heat and toxin, eliminate dampness.

Formula: Yin Qiao San (Honeysuckle and Forsythia Powder) and Liu Yi San (Six to One Powder) modified.

In the formula, Bo He (Herba Menthae Haplocalycis), Dan dou Chi (Semen Sojae Praeparatum) release the exterior. Jie Geng (Radix Platycodi Grandiflori) and Gan Cao (Radix Glycyrrhizae Uralensis) disperse the lungs and expel wind. Jin yin Hua (Flos Lonicerae Japonicae) and Lian Qiao (Rhizoma Coptidis) clear heat and toxin. Hua Shi (Talcum) and Che Qian Zi (Semen Plantaginis) clear heat and eliminate dampness.

Flaming heat in Qi and Ying

Manifestations

Persistent high fever, anxiety, thirst, dense and purple and reddish rashes, constipation, yellow urine, deep red tongue with thick and yellow coating, full and rapid pulse, stagnation of the index vein.

Treatment Principle Clear qi and cool the Ying, clear heat toxin and eliminate dampness.

Formula

Qing Wei Jie Du Tang(Clear Stomach and Removing Toxin Decoction)

Jin yin Hua (Flos Lonicerae Japonicae), Lian Qiao (Rhizoma Coptidis), Ban Lan Gen (Radix Isatidis Seu Baphicacanthi), Shi Gao (Gypsum), Huang Qin (Radix Scutellariae Baicalensis) clear heat and toxin. Sheng Di Huang (Radix Rehmanniae Glutinosae), Mu Dan Pi (Cortex Moutan Radicis) and Chi Shao (Radix Paeoniae Rubra) cool Ying, release toxin and activate blood. Dan Zhu Ye (Herba Loptatheri Gracilis) and Hua Shi (Talcum) clear heat and eliminate dampness. Qing Wen Bai Du Yin (Clear Epidemics and Overcome Toxin Decoction) is also used for this syndrome. If there is convultion and deliurum, add Zi Xue Dan (Purple Snow Special Pill), or An Gong Niu Huang Wan (Calm the Palace Pill with Cattle Gallstone) are recommended, as well as refer to appropriate MD.

Other Therapy

Patent herbs

- Ban Lang Gen Chong Ji (Radix Isatidis Seu Baphicacanthi Granule) taken orally 0.5~1bag per time, 3 times per day. It is used for pathogens stagnating in the lungs and Wei.
- Yin Qiao Wan (Honeysuckle and Forsythia Pills) taken orally 3~6g per time, 2 times a day. It is used for pathogens stagnating in the lungs and Wei.

Topical Therapy

Decoct Ku Shen (Radix Sophorae Flavescentis)30g, Mang Xiao (Mirabilite)30g and Fu Ping (Herba Spirodelae)15g, wash body with the herbal liquid. 2 times per day. It is used for dense rashes and itching.

Qing Dai (Indigo)5g mixed with Zhi Ma You (Sesame Oil) put on the local rashes. It is used for rashes that are broken.

Prevention and care

- Isolate patients until the scars of the blisters are gone.
- During the epidemic season, keep children away from public places.

- In patients who are taking steroids, immunosuppressants, or suffer from malignant diseases, shingles vaccination is recommended.
- Keep the skin clean and try to prevent skin infection.

Epidemic Encephalitis B
(Yi Xing Nao Yan乙性脑炎)

Epidemic Encephalitis B is an acute epidemic disease caused by a summer febrile pathogen and manifested by fever, loss of consciousness and convulsion. There were various names for the illness in ancient books: such as summer wind (Shu Feng), when main manifestation is shaking and jerking. Summer convulsion (Shu Jing), includes stiff neck or opisthotonos due to summer epidemic pathogen. Summer unconsciousness (Shu Jue), is cold extremities and sudden loss of consciousness due to summer epidemics attacking the pericardium. This correlated to epidemic encephalitis B in mainstream medicine. The chapter Shang Jiao in Wen Bing Tiao Bian (Detailed Analysis of Warm Diseases) points out "if children suffer from summer epidemic warm disease, manifested fever and sudden convulsion." Epidemic encephalitis is a disease caused by a virus infection. Mosquitoes are the main vector, it is transmitted through the bite of an infected mosquito and spread to humans and animals. Most of the population is susceptible to it with the majority of patients being under 10 years of age, and especially children 2 to 6 years old. After having the infection, people may get long-lasting immunity. The disease mostly spreads in the summer months. After the implementation of large-scale vaccination, the incidence rate is decreased significantly and it is mostly sporadic. It is an acute and critical issue. The prognosis of the mild case is a full recovery is possible. Severe cases can cause organ failure and can be fatal.

Etiology and pathology

The disorder is caused by summer febrile pathogen. Children's skin are soft, sparse barriers are thin with non-solid Wei Qi, Zang and Fu organs are delicate, their Qi and physique are immature; so children are susceptible to exterior pathogens. If they suffer febrile warm diseases, the pathogen will easily invade inside and tend to affect the Wei and Qi, or Qi and Ying, or even Qi, Ying and blood at the same time. Because the summer heat pathogen is violent, it tends to cause flaming fire, and generate phlegm, wind and convulsion. Moreover, the critical condition, the syndrome of interior closing and exterior exhaustion occurs very often. The summer heat tends to damage Qi and Yin. It causes the disease to linger at the late stage with the Qi and yin damaged and unresolved heat, phlegm and wind. The disabling sequela may occur if it lasts long term and damages Zang, Fu and meridians.

Pathogen invading the Wei and Qi Invasion of the Wei and disharmony of the exterior results in fever and slight aversion to cold. The pathogen swiftly turns into heat and fire, which transmits to the Yang Ming stage, resulting in high fever, thirst and constipation. The summer heat easily combines with dampness that causes fullness of the chest, vomiting, and lethargy due to damp heat retention in the Tai Yin and clouding the mind.

Flaming of pathogen in the Qi and Ying levels The pathogenic summer heat in the Qi level turns into fire which invades the Ying level. Excessive heat produces wind and phlegm, which blocks the heart orifice and stirs liver wind, causing high fever, unconsciousness and convulsion. The three syndromes of heat, phlegm and wind occur simultaneously.

Pathogen invading Ying and Blood levels The pathogen in the Ying and blood consumes yin, resulting in fever that is more pronounced at night. The mixed phlegm and heat clouds the heart orifice and stirs liver wind, which causes coma and repeated convulsions. The heat in the blood forces the abnormal movement of the blood, resulting in hematamesis, purple papules and rashes, The manifestations of collapse occurs, such as irregular breathing, pale complexion, severe cold extremities and very weak pulse due to high fever severely injuring Yuan Qi.

Vital Qi vacuity and pathogen lingering The complications and sequelae occur since pathogenic heat, phlegm and wind have stayed inside and have injured vital qi.

Yin vacuity due to Lingering heat Summer heat tends to injure yin. The pathogen lingers inside long term and consumes yin and body fluids, resulting in long-term low grade fever. It also may damage qi and cause disharmony between Ying and Wei, leading to an irregular fever for a long time.

Phlegm besieged the orifices Phlegm besieges the heart orifice, the root of the tongue, and the air passages, which results in unconsciousness, deafness, aphasia, gurgling in the throat, and dysphagia.

Internal wind stirring The heat lingers in the body, damages the liver and kidney yin. The yin fails to nourish the tendons, and lead to tremor and involuntary movement of the limbs. If the wind with phlegm clogging the meridians, it causes ankylosing paralysis.

Diagnosis

Diagnostic Guidelines

This most often occurs in the summer and autumn, but more commonly in July, August, and September. There are seasonal and environmental components to mosquito breeding patterns.

Manifestations

Patient may have fever, impaired consciousness manifested by irritability, drowsiness, stupor, or coma, seizures and/or status epilepticus, focal neurological dysfunction, stiff neck, malaise, nausea and vomiting.

Laboratory tests: Increased CSF protein, pressure, and CSF lymphocytic pleocytosis.

Differential of Diagnosis

Febrile convulsion These occur in children between 6 months and 3 years of age. Convulsions more commonly occur in the early stage of febrile diseases, and when the temperature suddenly spikes. The convulsions often last a couple of seconds or minutes. Conditions will commonly return to normal once the convulsions end. There is no repeated or continuous attacks, but often have previous history of seizures, and no neurological positive signs.

Epidemic Toxic Dysentery Severe dysentery marked by abrupt onset of high fever, convulsion and invisible(no bowel movement, no pus and bleeding in the bowel movement) or visible dysentery(loose bowel movement with pus and bleeding in feces). The closing and exhaustion syndrome easily occur, but generally no positive signs of meningeal irritation. Anal swab, or stool enema examination shows a lot of pus, white blood cells, and red blood cells.

Diagnostic Notes

- Pay attention to the epidemiological history.
- Note the characteristics of acute onset, and the changeable nature of disease.
- Observe the fever, unconsciousness, convulsion and the manifestations of internal closing and exterior exhaustion.
- Note the physical findings and signs of the nervous system.
- Check the ABC and NSF in time.

Pattern Differentiation

Guidelines of differentiation

- Differentiate between the mild and severe syndrome. If there is a persistent high fever, deep unconsciousness, frequent fits of convulsion, or the manifestations of interior closing and exterior exhaustion, it is the severe syndrome. Otherwise, it is mild.

- Differentiate between the syndromes of heat, phlegm and wind at the acute stage. If the pathogen is at the Wei level with symptoms of a heat syndrome, it is a heat syndrome. If the pathogen is at the Qi and Ying, or Ying and blood level with fever, unconsciousness and convulsion, it has the three syndromes of heat, phlegm and wind.
- Differentiate between the sequelae syndromes of heat, phlegm and wind in the recovery stage. If the heat stays inside but is not decreased manifesting a lower grade fever, it is heat syndrome. If there is unconsciousness, deafness, aphasia, gurgling in the throat and dysphagia due to phlegm besieged in the orifices. If there is tremors, involuntary movement of the limbs, and ankylosing paralysis, it is a wind syndrome due to interior wind stirring.

Therapeutic principle

Focus on clearing heat, dispelling phlegm, opening orifice, and extinguishing wind. Clearing heat from the Wei, Qi, Ying, and Blood is the main therapy at the acute stage and is according to which level the pathogen is located. Strengthening vital qi and expelling the pathogen is main therapy at the recovery stage. This consists of clearing heat and nourishing yin, dispelling phlegm and opening the orifices, and extinguishing wind and stopping convulsions.

Patterns and Treatment

Pathogen stagnating the lung and defensive level

Manifestations

Sudden fever, or mild chills, headache, thirst, nausea, vomiting, anxiety, or drowsiness, stiff neck, red tongue with thin and yellow coating. Floating and rapid pulse or full and rapid pulse. Floating and purple index finger vein.

Treatment Principle Relieve exterior with pungent and cool herbs, clear heat, and dispel toxin.

Formula

Yin Qiao San (Honeysuckle and Forsythia Powder) and Bai Hu Tang (White Tiger Decoction).

In the formula, Bo He (Herba Menthae Haplocalycis), Dan Dou Chi (Semen Sojae Praeparatum) and Ju Hua (Flos Chrysanthemi Morifolii) expel wind and release exterior. Jin Yin Hua (Flos Lonicerae Japonicae) and Lian Qiao (Rhizoma Coptidis), Ban Lan Gen (Radix Isatidis Seu Baphicacanthi), and Da Qing Ye (Folium Daqingye) clear heat and detoxify. He Ye (Nelumbo Nucifera) clears summer heat. Dan Zhu Ye (Herba Loptatheri Gracilis), and Lu Gen (Rhizoma Phragmitis Communis) clear heat and generate fluids. Shi Gao (Gypsum), Zhi Mu (Rhizome Anemarrhenae) clear heat and purge fire. If there is convulsion, add Chan Tui (Periostracum Cicadae) and Gou Teng (Ramulus Cum Uncis Uncariae). If the dampness is severe, add Xiang Ru (Herba Elsholtziae Seu Moslae), Huo Xiang (Herba Agastaches Seu Pogostemi), Pei Lan (Herba Eupatorii Fortunei) and Liu Yi San (Six to One Powder) to dispel dampness. If drowsiness is severe, add Shi Chang Pu (Rhizoma Acori Graminei) and Yu Jin (Tuber Curcumae) to eliminate dampness and open the orifice. If there is stiff neck, add Ge Gen (Radix Puerariae), Gou Teng (Ramulus Cum Uncis Uncariae) to extinguish wind and stop convulsion.

Flaming of heat in the Qi and Ying

Manifestations

Continuous high fever, thirst, severe headache, nausea, vomiting, restlessness, stiff neck, convulsion, gurgling in the throat, constipation, yellow urine, crimson tongue with dry and yellow coating, wiry and rapid pulse. Purple and stagnated pulse.

Treatment Principle Clear heat and cool Ying, dispel phlegm and stop convulsion.

Formula

Qing Wen Bai Du yin (Clear Epidemics and Overcome Toxin Decoction).

In the formula, Shi Gao (Gypsum), Zhi Mu (Rhizome Anemarrhenae) clear the heat in Qi level. Shui Niu Jiao (Cornu Bubali), Sheng Di Huang (Radix Rehmanniae Glutinosae), Mu Dan Pi (Cortex Moutan Radicis), and Chi Shao (Radix Paeoniae Rubra) clear heat toxin in the Ying level. Huang Qin (Radix Scutellariae Baicalensis), Huang Lian (Rhizoma Coptidis), Da Qing Ye (Folium Daqingye), Ban Lan Gen (Radix Isatidis Seu Baphicacanthi) clear heat and toxin. If there is repeated convulsion, also add Ling Yang Jiao (Antilope Horn), Gou Teng (Ramulus Cum Uncis Uncariae) and Di Long (Lumbricus) to calm the liver and extinguish wind. If there is unconsciousness, add An Gong Niu Huang Wan (Calm the Palace Pill with Cattle Gallstone).

Pathogen invading the Ying and Blood level

Manifestations

Unstable fever that is milder in the morning and worse in the night, unconsciousness, staring eyes, clenching mouth, frequent fits of convulsion, gurgling in the throat, hot trunk and cold limbs, or even purple maculae and bleeding, shortened tongue and crimson color, thin, rapid and wiry pulse. Purple index vein.

Treatment Principle Cool the blood and nourish yin, open orifice and extinguish wind.

Formula: Xi Jiao Di Huang Tang (Rhinoceros Horn and Rehmannia Decoction)

In the formula, Shui Niu Jiao (Cornu Bubali), and Sheng Di Huang (Radix Rehmanniae Glutinosae) clear ying and cool blood. Mu Dan Pi (Cortex Moutan Radicis) and Chi Shao (Radix Paeoniae Rubra) cool and invigorate blood, Xuan Shen (Radix Scrophulariae Ningpoensis) and Mai Men Dong (Tuber Ophiopogonis Japonici) clear heat and nourish Yin. If there is severe cold sweating, and a very deep and weak pulse, add Shen Fu Long Mu Jiu Ni Tang (Rescue Decoction of Ginseng, Prepared Aconite, Dragon Bone and Oyster Shell)

Yin vacuity due to Lingering heat

Manifestations

Long-term low grade fever, which is worse during the night, redness along the zygomatic arch, night sweating, anxiety, thirst, constipation, red tongue with less coating, thin and rapid pulse. Or irregular fever, pale complexion, tiredness, poor appetite, cloose stool, pale tongue with thin, white coating, thread pulse.

Treatment Principle Nourish yin and clear heat. Strengthen Qi and relieve heat.

Formula

Qing Hao Bie Jia Tang (Sweet Wormwood and Turtle Shell Decoction), or Huang Qi Gui Zhi Wu Wu Tang (Astragalus and Cinnamon Twig Five-Substance Decoction).

In the formula, Bie Jia(Turtle Shell) nourishes Yin and relieves heat. Qing Hao (Sweet Wormwood) expels the heat out. Sheng Di Huang (Radix Rehmanniae Glutinosae), Mu Dan Pi (Cortex Moutan Radicis), and Zhi Mu (Rhizome Anemarrhenae) nourish Yin, clear heat, and cool blood. If there is more night sweating, also add Bai shao (Radix Paeoniae Lactiflorae) and Wu Wei Zi (Fructus Schisandrae Chinensis) to bind yin and stop sweating. If thirst, add Shi Hu (Dendrobium Stem) and Tian Hua Fen (Radix Trichosanthes) to nourish yin and generate fluids. If jerky movement, add Shi Jue Ming (Concha Haliotidis) and Zhen Zhu Mu (Margarita) to sedate yang and extinguish wind. If the fever is due to disharmony between Ying and Wei, use Huang Qi Gui Zhi Wu Wu Tang (Astragalus and Cinnamon Twig Five-Substance Decoction).

Phlegm obstructing the orifices

Manifestations

Cloudy mind, unconsciousness, deafness, aphasia, gurgling in the throat, dysphagia, red tongue with greasy coating. Slippery pulse.

Treatment Principle Scour out the phlegm, opens up the orifices.

Formula

Di Tan Tang Scours out the phlegm, opens up the orifices and supplements the Qi.

In the formula, Ban Xia (Rhizoma Pinelliae Ternatae), Chen Pi (Pericarpium Citri Reticulatae), Fu Ling (Sclerotium Poria Cocos) resolve phlegm and regulate Qi. Zhi Shi (Fructus Immaturus Citri Aurantii) scours out phlegm and open the chest. Shi Chang Pu (Rhizoma Acori Graminei) and Yu Jin (Tuber Curcumae) eliminate phlegm, Yuan Zhi (Radix Polygalae Tenuifoliae) eliminates phlegm and opens orifices. Dan Nan Xing (Arisaema Consanguineum Prepared with Bile) and Zhu Ru (Caulis Bambusae in Taeniis) clear heat and expel phlegm. If there is unconsciousness with white and greasy coating, add Su He Xiang Wang (Liquid Styrax Pill).

Internal wind stirring

Manifestations

Tremor and involuntary movements of limbs, or ankylosing paralysis, crimson tongue with a peeled coating, thin, wiry, and rapid pulse.

Treatment Principl: Extinguish wind and stop tremor.

Formula

Da Ding Feng Zhu Major Arrest Wind Pearls)

In the formula, Ji Zi Huang (Egg Yolk) one, E Jiao (Colla Corii Asini) nourish Yin. Di Huang (Radix Rehmanniae Glutinosae), Xuan Shen (Radix Scrophulariae Ningpoensis) and Mai Men Dong (Tuber Ophiopogonis Japonici), and Bai shao (Radix Paeoniae Lactiflorae) nourish Yin and generate fluid. Gui Ban (Plastrum Testudinis) and Bie Jia (Fresh-water Turtle Shell) nourish Yin and sedate Yang. Zhen Zhu Mu (Margarita) and Mu Li (Concha Ostreae) sedate Yang and extinguish wind. If there is profuse sweating, weakness, fatigue, poor appetite and pale complexion, add Huang Qi (Astragalus), Dang Shen (Radix Codonopsitis Pilosulae) and Shan Yao (Radix Dioscoreae Oppositae) to strengthen the spleen and stomach.

Other Therapy

Patent herbs

- Niu Huang Qian Jin San (Bezoar Thousand Ducat Powder) taken orally 0.5~0.6g per time, 2 times per day. It is used for pathogens in the Qi and Ying levels.
- Shen Xi Dan Oral taking 3g per time, 2 times per day. It is used for pathogen in the Ying and blood.

Acupuncture

- Puncture Du26, Yintang, Du14, LI11, LI4, GB34, Liv3. Strong reducing, and bleeding Sixuan, 2~3 times per day. It is used for high fever, coma and convulsion due to pathogen in the Qi and Ying.
- Puncture Du26, Du14, UB12, PC6, Ht7, St40. Once a day. It is used for anxiety due to heat phlegm obstructing the orifices during the recovery stage.
- Puncture Ren22, Ren23, LI4, St44. Once a day. It is used for deafness due to phlegm obstructing the orifices during the recovery stage.
- Puncture Du16, Ren23, Ht5, LI4, Ki6, Ki1. Once a day. It is used for dysphagia due to phlegm obstructing the orifices during the recovery stage.

- Puncture LI15, LI11, SJ5, LI4, GB30, GB31, GB34, St36, UB40, GB40, UB62 once a day. It is used for stiffness of limbs.
- Puncture Du14, LI10, PC5, LI4, GB34, GB39 once a day. It is used for tremor due to wind stirring up during the recovery stage.

Tuina

It is used for sequela of the stiff joints and limbs paralysis during the recovery stage.

Prevention and care

- Patients should reduce exposure to mosquitoes by using repellents, protective clothing, and insecticede
- Patients should avoid behaviors that increase the risk of herpes virus or HIV infection
- Patients should avoid environments where causative viral agents and their vectors are endemic
- Closely observe respiration, pulse, blood pressure, pupils and other changes in the patient.
- Travelers to rural areas and mosquito-prone areas during the summer months should consider a newly available vaccine against Japanese B encephalitis

Epidemic Toxic Dysentery (Yu Du Li 疫毒痢)

Epidemic Toxic Dysentery is a severe and critical dysentery manifested with abrupt onset of high fever, unconsciousness, convulsion, and invisible, or visible dysentery, and even the syndrome of interior closed and exterior exhausted. It is also known as abrupt dysentery, or heat and toxic dysentery. It is named as toxic bacillary dysentery in Western medicine. Patients and carriers of the bacteria are the source of infection. The pathogen is in food, water, and on hands of infected people and is transmitted through the mouth. It occurs in summer and fall, in children under 2~7 years old. Since it is critical and mortality is high, it is important to make a diagnosis at the early stage of the disease so that treatment will not be delayed.

Etiology and pathology

It is caused by epidemic damp toxin invading the intestines and stomach due to the insufficient intestines and stomachs in children. Since the Yang pathogen lodges in the intestine and stomach, it causes necrosis of the intestine and stomach, changes it into pus, and also turns into fire abruptly.

Heat toxin closing the Interior The invasion of heat-toxin in the stomach and intestine abruptly turns into fire, and penetrates into the Jueyin, interiorly closes the heart orifice, which leads to high fever, unconsciousness, convulsion.

The syndrome of interior closed and exterior exhausted Since the heat toxin is an extreme excess and the body Qi is too weak to defend against the pathogen, the result is heat toxin closing interiorly, while Yang Qi collapses abruptly at the exterior. This is manifested with pale complexion, cold extremities with sweating, weak breath and a very deep pulse.

Diagnosis

Diagnostic Guidelines

Epidemiological history This occurs more in the summer and fall. The disease spreads within the same area. The children have a recent history of eating contaminated food, or exposure to a patient who has dysentery.

Manifestations and signs

Abrupt onset of high fever, unconsciousness, convulsion, and invisible, or visible dysentery, even the syndrome of closed and exterior exhausted. Diarrhea with pus doesn't show first in most of the patients, feces with pus and blood is found by enema.

279

Laboratory Exam

WBC count may be increased, primarily neutrophils.

Culture: there is growth of <u>E. coli</u> for 6~8 hours.

Diagnostic Notes

- Pay attention the history of epidemics
- Note the characters of acute onset, abruptly changeable of disease
- Observe the fever, unconsciousness, convulsions and the manifestations of internal closing and exterior exhaustion
- Stool samples are taken for examination under a microscope and for a laboratory culture to confirm the presence of the *shigella bacillus*.

Pattern Differentiation

Differentiation of Diagnosis

Febrile convulsion: Please refer to the differentiation of diagnosis of epidemic encephalitis B

Epidemic encephalitis B: The high fever, unconsciousness and convulsion epidemic encephalitis B often occurs in 2~3 days after onset. The syndrome of exterior exhaustion is not so common. It hardly shows dehydration. The focal neurological dysfunction, stiff neck and unconsciousness occurs. It also has increased CSF protein, pressure, and CSF lymphocytic pleocytosis.

Guidelines of differentiation

Differentiate between the mild and severe interior closed syndrome: If the fever is mild, short and infrequent convulsions, mild unconsciousness, and there is dysenteric feces, it suggests the interior closed syndrome is mild. If the patient has a high fever, frequent convulsions with long duriation, and deep coma, it is a severe case.

Differentiate between the mild and severe syndrome of exterior exhaustion: If there is a pale complexion, cold limbs, mild purple lips and skin, a slightly lowered blood pressure; it is a mild case of exterior exhaustion. If there is green and purple complexion and lips, very cold limbs and sweating, bleeding, no urine, uneven depth and rhythm of breathing, very deep and weak pulse, very low blood pressure, it is the severe syndrome of exterior exhaustion.

Therapeutic Principle

The disease must be actively treated to clear heat and toxin, open the closed and bind the exhaustion. If it is due to the syndrome of interior closed by heat toxin, then purging fire, opening closed syndrome, and preventing exterior exhaustion is recommended. If it is due to Yang exhausted in the exterior, rescuing yang from danger and preventing abrupt depletion of yang, it is necessary to refer these patients to an MD.

Patterns and Treatment

Syndrome of heat toxin closing interior

Manifestations

Abrupt high fever, dry lips, thirst, nausea and vomiting, anxiety and delirium, even coma, convulsion, scanty urine, or dysentery with pus and blood, or feces with pus and blood found with enema. Red tongue with thick yellow coating, and slippery and rapid pulse.

Treatment Principle Clear heat and relieve toxin, purge fire and open the closed syndrome.

Formula

Bai Tou Weng Tang(pulstilla decoction)
    In the formula, Huang Bai (Cotex Phellodendri), Huang Lian (Rhizoma Coptidis), Huang Qin (Radix Scutellariae Baicalensis),

and Qin Pi (Cortex Fraxini) clear heat, purge fire and relieve toxin. Da Huang (Radix et Rhizoma Rhei), and Zhi Shi (Unripened Bitter Orange) eliminate toxin by purging. Bai Tou Weng (Pulstilla), Ma Chi Xian (Portulaca Oleracea), and Di Yu (Radix Sanguisorbae Officinalis) clear heat, cool blood and are anti-dysentery herbs. If the vomiting is severe, also add Gou Teng (Ramulus Cum Uncis Uncariae) and Di Long (Lumbricus) to clear heat and extinguish wind. If there is a clouded mind, add Shi Chang Pu, and Yu Jin (Tuber Curcumae) to eliminate phlegm and wake up the mind. If there is coma, add Zi Xue Dan (Purple Snow Special Pill), or An Gong Niu Huang Wan (Calm the Palace Pill with Cattle Gallstone) to open the orifice and wake up the spirit.

Syndrome of interior closed and exterior exhaustion

Manifestations

The manifestations of the syndrome of interior closed are high fever, coma, convulsion, sudden fever drops, profuse cold sweat, pale complexion and skin, cold limbs, less urine or no urine, uneven depth and rhythm of breathing, very deep and weak pulse, very low blood pressure, and pale index finger vein.

Treatment Principle Strengthen yang qi, rescue the collapsing state.

Formula

Shen Fu Long Mu Jiu Ni Tang (Rescue Decoction of Ginseng, Prepared Aconite, Dragon Bone and Oyster Shell)

First use Ren Shen (Radix Ginseng), and Fu Zi (Radix Aconiti Carmichaeli) to strengthen Yang Qi and rescue the collapsing state. If it is a severe case, add Long Gu (Os Draconis), Mu Li (Concha Ostreae), Bai Shao (Radix Paeoniae Lactiflorae) and Gan Cao (Radix Glycyrrhizae Uralensis) to strengthen the functions of sedating the Yang and rescuing the collapsing state. If there are purple lips and skin, also add Dang Gui (Radix Angelicae Sinensis), Tao Ren (Semen Persicae), Hong Hua (Flos Carthami Tinctorii) and Chi Shao (Radix Paeoniae Rubra). If there is uneven depth and rhythm of breathing, add Wu Wei Zi (Fructus Schisandrae Chinensis) and Shan Zhu Yu (Fructus Corni Officinalis) to bind the lungs and kidney.

Acupuncture treatment

- Strongly stimulate Du26, Yintang, Du14, LI11, LI4, PC6, Liv3, St36. 2-3times per day. It is used for the syndrome of heat toxin closed interior
- Puncture Du26, Ht8, moxa Du20, Ren8, Ren6. 2~3 times per day. It is used for the syndrome of interior closed and exterior exhausted.

Prevention and Care

To prevent the spread of infection, keep the toilet clean and wash your hands frequently with warm water and soap, especially after a bowel movement or before handling food.

When traveling abroad or in areas with poor sanitation, drink only bottled or boiled water or other bottled beverages, and eat only cooked foods and fruit you can peel yourself.

Avoid contact with infected people if possible.

Infectious Mononucleosis
(Chuan Ran Xing Dan He Xi Bao Zeng
Duo Zheng 传染性单核细胞增多症)

Infectious mononucleosis (IM), also known as Mono is an infectious, widespread viral disease caused by the Epstein–Barr virus (EBV) manifested with fever, sore throat, swollen lymph nodes, swollen liver and spleen and increased atypical lymphocytes. Most people are exposed to the virus as children when the disease produces no noticeable or only flu-like symptoms. In developing countries, people are exposed to the virus in early childhood more often than in developed countries. It is most common among adolescents and young adults. Epstein–Barr virus infection is spread via saliva, and has an incubation period of four to seven weeks. Some studies indicate that a person can spread the infection for many months, possibly up to a year and a half. The prognosis of the disease is mostly good with the treatment. Serious complications are uncommon. There is no name of the disease in ancient Chinese medical literature, but there are diseases with similar symptoms described. For example "The febrile toxin leading to sore throat and swollen tonsils, and also swelling behind the ears *in Wen Bing Tiao Bian* (Detailed Analysis of Warm Diseases). According to the manifestations, it may be differentiated with febrile warm diseases.

Etiology and pathology

The disorder is due to the invasion of exterior febrile pathogens that affects the lungs, and the pathogen transfers to the Wei, Qi, Ying and Blood level.

Pathogens invading the lungs and stomach The febrile pathogen first invades the lungs, and stagnates in the lungs and Wei level, resulting in manifestations of the Wei level, such as fever and chills, headache and cough, reddish and painful throat. The pathogen also attacks the stomach, causing reversal stomach Qi, resulting in nausea, vomiting and poor appetite. If there is dampness with it, patients may have a heavy sensation of the body, fullness of the chest and abdomen.

Flaming of heat at Qi and Ying The pathogen has not been relieved at the Wei level, it transfers into qi and Ying, the heat flames the qi and Ying, and burns the body fluids, phlegm and heat accumulates together. This results in high fever, thirst, swollen lymph nodes, and swollen liver and spleen. If the phlegm heat closes the lungs, it results in cough, shortness of breath, and nasal flaring. If heat toxin with dampness stagnates in the liver and gallbladder, it may cause jaundice. If heat toxin disturbs the Ying and Blood, it may force blood to move faster than normal resulting in purpura. If the heat toxin invades the heart and liver, it may cause coma and convulsion. If the pathogen blocks the meridian, it results in deviation of the eyes and mouth, aphonia, and paralysis of the limbs.

Vacuity both qi and yin The heat lingers inside the body and damages qi and qin, which results in low grade fever, fatigue, thirst, and hot flashes.

Diagnosis

Diagnostic Guidelines

Epidemiological history: Incubation period is 5~15 days in childhood. There are preclinical symptoms, such as fatigue, headache, dizziness, poor appetite, nausea, vomiting, and slight diarrhea.

Manifestations and signs

Irregular fever, the temperature is from 101.3F° to 104F°, or with chills, and it may last 4~5 weeks. Most of the lymph nodes inside body are swollen, sore throat with swollen tonsils, or with bleeding and ulcers in throat. Splenohepatomegaly that is tender to palpation. There are papules and maculae on the skin. If the lungs, kidney, heart and brain are damaged, cough, hematuria, convulsion and paralysis may occur.

Laboratory Exam: WBC count increased to 10 to 20 $\times$ 10 9 / L or more, Lymphocytes and monocytes increased, more than 50%. Atypical lymphocytes>10%. IgG, when positive, reflects a past infection, whereas IgM reflects a current infection. Specific blood tests, such as the monospot and heterophile antibody tests, can confirm the diagnosis of Mono.

Differentiation of Diagnosis

Streptococcal pharyngitis: includes sore throat, temperature greater than 100.4°F (38°C), tonsillar exudates, and cervical adenopathy. Strep bacteria can be obtained by swabbing the back of the throat or the rectum with a piece of sterile cotton. Microscopic examination of the smear can identify which type of bacteria has been collected.

Infectious lymphocytosis: manifested with mild fever, swollen lymph nodes and spleen, increase in the number or proportion of lymphocytes in the blood and elevated total lymphocyte count.

Diagnostic Notes

Note the relationship between the fever and swollen lymph nodes, and pay attention to the history of exposure to epidemic diseases.

Palpate for lymph nodes become enlargement in locations, such as the neck and the medial epicondyle. Pay attention to the size, texture, tenderness, and the presence or absence of adhesions of the nodes. Also palpate the liver and spleen.

Pattern Differentiation

Guidelines of differentiation

Differentiate between the mild and severe syndrome: If the pathogen is at the Wei and Qi level it manifests with fever, sore throat, swollen lymph nodes, no swelling the spleen and liver, it is a mild syndrome. If the pathogen is in the Qi and Ying or Blood level it is manifested with pneumonia, jaundice and convulsion due to high fever, and it is considered the severe syndrome.

Differentiate between the stage of the disease, repletion and vacuity: If the disease is at the early and middle stages, the pathogen is in Wei, Qi and Ying level accompanied with dampness, blood stasis, and phlegm, it is a repletion syndrome. If it is in the later stage, body fluids and Qi are consumed with pathogen lingering, it is due to vacuity, or combined repletion and vacuity.

Therapeutic principle

The treatment principle is to clear heat and relieve toxin, eliminate phlegm and quicken blood. If the pathogen is in the Wei level, add the method of expelling wind and relieving exterior. If it is in the Qi level, purge heat. If the pathogen is in the Ying and Blood, cool the blood. If it is late stage, nourish the yin and strengthen Qi.

Pathogen stagnating in the lungs and stomach

Manifestations

Fever, mild chills, reddish and painful throat, painful swollen lymph nodes, poor appetite, nausea and vomiting, loose stool, red tongue with thin and yellow coating, floating and rapid pulse.

Treatment Principle Clear heat and relieve toxin, disperse the lungs and sooth the throat.

Formula

Yin Qiao San (Honeysuckle and Forsythia Powder).

In the formula, Bo He (Herba Menthae Haplocalycis), Jin Yin Hua (Flos Lonicerae Japonicae) and Lian Qiao (Rhizoma Coptidis) clear heat and toxin. Niu Bang Zi (Fructus Arctii), Jie Geng (Radix Platycodi Grandiflori) disperse the lungs and sooth throat. Lu Gen (Rhizoma Phragmitis Communis) and Dan Zhu Ye (Herba Loptatheri Gracilis) clear heat and generate fluids. Add Ban Lan Gen (Radix Isatidis Seu Baphicacanthi) and Xuan Shen (Radix Scrophulariae Ningpoensis) clear heat and toxin. Also add Huo Xiang (herba Agastaches seu Pogostemi), Ban Xia (Rhizoma Pinelliae Ternatae), Fu Ling (Sclerotium Poria Cocos) to harmonize the stomach and eliminate dampness.

Flaming of heat at Qi and Ying

Manifestations

Persistent high fever, thirst, reddish and painful throat possible with pus, swollen lymph nodes, swollen liver and spleen, and purple macules. Red tongue with yellow coating, full and rapid pulse.

Treatment Principle Clear heat and cool the Ying, relieve toxin and soothe the throat.

Formula

Qing Wen Bai Du yin (Clear Epidemics and Overcome Toxin Decoction).

In the formula, Zhi Mu (Rhizome anemarrhenae), Shui Niu Jiao (Cornu Bubali), Sheng Di Huang (Radix Rehmanniae Glutinosae), Mu Dan Pi (Cortex Moutan Radicis), and Chi Shao (Radix Paeoniae Rubra) clear heat and toxin in the Ying. Huang Qin (Radix Scutellariae Baicalensis), Huang Lian(Rhizoma Coptidis), Zhi Zi (Fructus Gardeniae Jasminoidis), Da Qing Ye (Folium Daqingye) clear heat and toxins. Also add She Gan (Belamcanda Chinesis), Xuan Shen (Radix Scrophulariae Ningpoensis) to clear heat and soothe the throat. If there are swollen lymph nodes, add Xiao Lou Wan (Reduce Scrofula Pill). If there is jaundice, swollen liver and spleen, add Yin Chen Hao Tang (Retenisia Yinchenhao Decoction). If there is pneumonia, add Ma Xing Shi Gan Tang (Ephedra, Apricot, Licorice and Gypsum Decoction). If there is convulsion and unconsciousness, add Ling Yang Gou Teng Tang (Antelope Horn and Uncaria Decoction).

Qi vacuity and pathogen lingering

Manifestations

Chronic course of disease, faded fever or low grade fever, fatigue, thirst, scanty urine, constipation, the swollen lymph nodes and the enlarged liver becomes smaller, red tongue with less coating, thin and weak pule.

Treatment Principle Nourish the yin, strengthen qi, clear lingering heat, unblock meridians, and invigorate blood.

Formula

Qing Hao Bie Jia Tang (Sweet Wormwood and Soft-Shelled Turtle Shell Decoction)

In the formula, Qing Hao (Sweet Wormwood), Bie Jia (Soft-Shelled Turtle Shell), Sheng Di Huang (Rehmannia Root), Mu

Dan Pi (Moutan Bark), Zhi Mu (Anemarrhena Rhizome) nourish Yin and clear heat. If there is constipation, also add Gua Lou Ren (Semen Trichosanthis) to moisten the intestines. If there is poor appetite, add Mai Ya (Fructus Hordei Vulgaris Germinantus) and Gu Ya (Fructus Oryzae Sativae Germinantus) to help digestion. If there are long-term swollen lymph nodes, add Xiao Lou Wan (Reduce Scrofula Pill) to relieve phlegm and soften masses. If there is splenohepatomegaly, add Yu Jin (Tuber Curcumae) and Dan Shen (Radix Salviae Miltiorrhizae) to invigorate blood.

Other Therapy

Patent herbs

- An Gong Niu Huang Wan(Calm the Palace Pill with Cattle Gallstone): For under 3 years old, oral taking ¼ pill per time. For 4 years old, ½ pill per time. 3 times per day. It is used for pathogens in the liver and heart.
- Sheng Mai yin (Generate the pulse liquid): taken orally, 5~10ml per time, 3 times per day. It is used for Qi and Yin vacuity at the late stage.

Acupuncture

- For fever. Du14, LI11, LI4, SJ5. Purging technique, no needle retention.
- For heat and blood stasis in the liver and gallblader. Du14, Sp9, Liv3, LI4 and LI11. If there is swollen liver and rib-side pain, add Liv13, and SJ6. Purging technique, keep needles retained for 20~30minutes.

Tui Na

Clear the lung channel and Tian He Shui, open Tian Men, transform Tai Yang, push Kan Gong, Tui Liu Fu.

Topical therapy

- Ru Yi Jin Huang San(Wish Fullfilling Golden Yellow) mixed with Tea or vinegar, apply on the swollen lymph nodes, twice a day.
- Xi Lou Wan(Resolving Nodules Pill): puff it on the throat, 3 times a day.

Prevention and Care

- Get plenty of rest for about 1~3 weeks to recover. Patients may need bed rest at the acute stage
- Gargle with salt water or use throat lozenges to soothe the sore throat
- Avoid contact sports and heavy lifting. The spleen may be enlarged, and impact or straining could cause it to burst
- Avoid thick and greasy foods

Parasitosis
(Ji Sheng Chong Bing 寄生虫病)

Parasitosis includes protozoal diseases and worm diseases. There are nine kinds of parasitosis in ancient Chinese medical literature. The roundworm and pinworm are the most prevenlent and harmful to the health of children in the clinic. Roundworm and pinworm parasitically stay in the intestines, which directly impacts the function of the stomach and intestines, consuming the essence from food, weakening the vital qi and disturbing the body's spirit. The roundworm may also travel through the biliary track and even into the gallbladder, or block the intestines causing a critical condition. Ancient physicians knew about some of parasites and they are mentioned in the Yellow Emperor's Classic, and the information is useful today.

Ascariasis (Hui Chong Bing 蛔虫病)

Ascariasis is a disease caused by the parasitic roundworm Ascaris lumbricoides living in the intestine, manifesting with pain around the umbilicus. The category of Parasitosis includes protozoal diseases and worm diseases. There were nine kinds of parasites in ancient Chinese medical literature. The roundworm and pinworm are the most prevalent and harmful to the health of children in the clinic. Roundworm and pinworm parasitically stay in the intestines, which directly impacts the function of the stomach and intestines, consuming the essence of food, weakening the vital qi and disturbing the body's spirit. The roundworm may also travel through the biliary tree and even into the gallbladder, or block the intestines causing a critical condition. Ancient physicians knew of some of the parasites and were mentioned in the Yellow Emperor's Classic, and their information is useful today. Intermittently and randomly, roundworm eggs can be found in the feces. If it becomes chronic, there may be poor appetite, dull complexion and can ultimately affect the child's development. The manifestations were mentioned in *the Huang Di Nei Jing* (The Yellow Emperor's Classic of TCM). In the chapter on cough it states "the stomach cough manifests with cough and vomiting, even severe vomiting of round worms". In *the Huang Di Nei Jing* chapter on Jue (Syncope with cold extremities) syndrome it states "The worms in the intestine may also cause worm blockage in the intestine manifesting with pain in the heart and intestines, masses that may move up or down, intermittent and unpredictable pain, hotness at the abdomen, thirst with salivation." The disease occurs year round, and children are more commonly affected. The incidence of roundworm is higher in rural areas.

Etiology and pathology

The main cause of ascariasis occurs by consuming fecal contaminated food or drink containing the *Ascaris* eggs. The eggs hatch in the intestines, burrow through the gut wall, and migrate to the lungs via the blood. There they break into the alveoli and pass up the trachea, where they are coughed up and swallowed. The larvae then pass through the stomach into the intestine where they become adult worms.

Ascariasis due to parasites in the intestines The roundworm that stays in the intestines disturbs the Qi function of the stomach and intestines, resulting in abdominal pain. If it affects the function of ascending and descending of qi, it causes stomach qi to be rebellious, there will be nausea, vomiting, profuse salivation, and poor appetite. If the roundworms stay in the intestine, this generates damp-heat, which accumulates in the spleen, the spleen and stomach are disharmonious, causing an addiction to eating abnormal things, nose itching, and pale spots on the face. The roundworms also consume the essence of food and produce toxin, which damages the spleen and stomach. The spleen and stomach fail to transform and transport. This weakens the qi and blood, manifesting with poor appetite, dull complexion, fatigue, and poor development. This is called Roundworm Gan (malnutrition due to roundworm).

Roundworm Jue (cold extremities) Syndrome Roundworms tend to enter the holes of organs or orifices. They travel through the biliary track and into the gallbladder causing Jue syndrome, which manifests with severe abdominal pain and cold extremities. These symptoms are similar to acute cholangitis or acute cholecystitis in Western medicine.

Roundworm mass syndrome The worms can occasionally cause intestinal blockage when large numbers get tangled into a bolus or more explanation, and may manifest with severe abdominal pain, vomiting and constipation, which is named roundworm mass. If infected by roundworms in a short time, they may travel through many organs, and cause related organ diseases, such as inflammation of the lungs, visceral damage, peritonitis, and inflammation and enlargement of the liver or spleen. Ascariasis may also result in allergies to shrimp and dust mites.

Diagnosis

Diagnostic Guidelines

Pain around the umbilicus that appears intermittently and unpredictably, addiction to eating abnormal objects, weight loss, the presence of roundworms or eggs in the feces.

Differentiation of Diagnosis

Abdominal pain due to food stagnation

The pain is in the upper abdomen and stomach area, which is worse when it is pressed. The pain is less after bowel movement containing undigested food. The patient has a history of over-eating.

Abdominal pain due to cold

The pain comes on suddenly, and it is relieved by warmth. There is bowel movement with loose stool and poor appetite.

Diagnostic Notes

- Inquire if there is a history of eating contaminated food or drink
- Inquire if there is vomitus containing roundworms, and the typical symptoms of sudden abdominal pain, or a preference for eating abnormal things
- Palpate the abdomen carefully to determine the location and characteristics of the pain. Test the stool for the presence of roundworm eggs.

Pattern Differentiation

Guidelines of Differentiation

- Differentiate between the various locations of the abdomen. If there is pain around the umbilicus that appears intermittently and unpredictably, the abdomen feels rope-like in the intestine with mild pain on palpation, it is roundworms in the intestine. If the pain is in the upper right abdominal quadrant, comes on suddenly, with episodes of severe colic, pain is worse when pressed, it is roundworm Jue (cold extremities) syndrome. If the pain is around umbilicus and there are streaks in the abdomen when palpated, it is a roundworm mass.
- Differentiating the severity of the syndrome. If the pain is mild and of short duration, it is a mild syndrome. If the pain is severe and lasts a long time, it is likely roundworm Jue (cold extremities) syndrome or roundworm mass and which is a severe syndrome.

Therapeutic principle

The basic principle is to calm the roundworm and stop pain, expel and kill roundworm, and strengthen the spleen and stomach. If there is severe abdominal pain, first calm the roundworm to stop pain, then expel and kill the roundworm, then strengthen the spleen and stomach. Roundworm has the following characteristics: it is calmed by sour herbs, it hides from pungent herbs, and is purged by bitter herbs. The formula should contain herbs with all of these flavors.

Patterns and treatment

Roundworm syndrome

Manifestations

No symptoms or only mild symptoms, occasional abdominal pain that is around the umbilicus. The pain appears intermittently and unpredictably, poor appetite, nausea, profuse salivation, addiction to eating abnormal objects, such as soil, teas, or charcoal. There may be anxiety, restlessness, and itchy nose. There also may be dull complexion, fatigue, irregular bowel movements, abdominal fullness, and weight loss. The tongue may have a greasy or peeled coating, and there may be pale spots on the tongue.

Treatment principle Expel and kill roundworm, and strengthen the spleen and stomach.

Formula

Shi Jun Zi San(Quisqualis Powder)
   In the formula, Shi Jun Zi (Fructus Quisqualis), Wu Yi (Fructus Ulmi), and Chuan Lian Zi (Fructus Toosendan) expel and kill roundworms. If there is abdominal fullness and constipation, add Da Huang (Radix et Rhizoma Rhei) and Bing Lang (Semen Arecae) to regulate Qi and stop pain. If there is poor appetite and vomiting, add Ban Xia (Rhizoma Pinelliae Terntae), Chen Pi (Pericarpium

Citri Reticulatae) and Shan Zha (frutus crataegi) to strengthen the spleen and stomach and harmonize the stomach. If there is fatigue and weight loss, add Yi Gong San (Extraodinary Merit Powder) to strengthen the spleen and stomach.

Roundworm Jue Syndrome

Manifestations

In addition to the above manifestations, there will be severe abdominal pain, which is in the stomach area or under right rib-side region, nausea, vomiting, or vomitus containing roundworms, chills, sweating, jaundice, tongue with a yellow greasy coating, wiry and rapid pulse.

Treatment principle First calm roundworms and stop pain, then expel worms.

Formula

Wu Mei Wan (Mume Fruit Pill)
   In the formula, Wu Mei (Fructus Pruni Mume) calms roundworms and stops pain. Huang Bai (Cotex Phellodendri), Huang Lian (rhizoma coptidis), Gan Jiang (Rhizoma Zingiberis), Xi Xin (Herba cun Radicae Asari) descend Qi to harmonize the middle and stop vomiting. Chuan Jiao (Si Chuan Pepper), Fu Zi (Radix Aconiti Carmichaeli) warm the middle and calms roundworms. Dang Shen (Radix Codonopsitis Pilosulae) and Dang Gui (Radix angelicae sinesis) supplement Qi and blood. If there is jaundice and a tongue with a yellow greasy coating, subtract Fu Z i(Radix Aconiti Carmichaeli), Gan Jiang (Rhizoma Zingiberis), Xi Xin (Herba Cun Radicae Asari), add Da Huang (Radix et Rhizoma Rhei), Yin Chen Hao (Herba Artemisiae Yinchenhao) and Huang Qin (Radix Scutellariae Baicalensis. If there is severe pain, add Zhi Ke (Peel of Fructus Immaturus Citri Aurantii), Da Huang (Radix et Rhizoma Rhei), and Yan Hu Suo (Corydalis Yanhusuo). After the pain is relieved, Shi Jun Zi San (Quisqualis Powder) is recommended.

Roundworm mass syndrome

Manifestations

The patient has history of ascariasis. Sudden onset of severe abdominal pain and abdominal fullness, frequent vomiting which may contain roundworms, constipation, masses, or a rope-like feeling in the intestine when palpated, tongue with a white or yellow greasy coating, slippery and rapid pulse.

Treatment principle Regulate qi and stop pain, resolve roundworm mass and expel worm.

Formula

Da Cheng Qi Tang (Major Order Qi Decoction) and Shi Jun Zi San (Quisqualis Powder).

In the formula, Da Huang (Radix et Rhizoma Rhei) purges heat in the stomach and intestines. Mang Xiao (Mirabilite) helps Da Huang soften masses, Hou Po (Cotex Magnoliae Officinalis) and Zhi Shi (Fructus Immaturus Citri Aurantii) regulate qi, unblock streaks and reduce abdominal fullness. Shi Jun Zi San (Quisqualis Powder) expels and kills roundworm.

Other Therapy

Patent herbs

- Wu Mei Wan (Mume Fruit Pill) Taken orally 3g T.I.D. It is used for roundworm Jue Syndrome due to co-mingling of heat and cold.
- Hua Chong Wan (Dissolve Parasites Pill) Taken orally 5g T.I.D. It is used for ascariasis due to damp heat.
- Fei Er Wan (Fat Baby Pill) Taken orally 1g T.I.D. It is used for malnutrition due to ascariasis.

Acupuncture

- To relax spasm and stop pain: Puncture St25, Ren12, St36, GB34 and PC6. Strongly stimulate for 3-5 minutes.
- To expel worms Puncture Sp15 (Towards to Ren8), St36, SJ6 with strong stimulation to purge the roundworm. Perform twice a day.
- For Roundworm Jue Syndrome Puncture St4 towards LI20 and puncture GB34. Strongly stimulate the needles. Retain the needles 20 minutes

Tuina

This is used for abdominal pain due to roundworm without high fever, jaundice. After massage put Hua Shi (Tacum) on the abdomen, then the practitioner uses the palm of his hand on the child's umbilicus, and kneads it clockwise.

Topical therapy

Grad Ku Lian Gen Pi (Peel of Melia Toosendan)200g, Cong Bai (Onions)100g, Hu Jiao (White Peper)20 pieces, fry them with vinegar 150ml, wrap them and warm the UB channel on the back from upper to lower repeatedly. It is used for abdominal pain due to roundworm. You may also mix Da Huang (Radix et Rhizoma Rhei)45g, Mang Xiao (Mirabilitum)45g and Bing Pian (Borneol)15g with vinegar, and put them on the abdomen.

Prevention and care

- Primary preventive measures include clean sanitary conditions, good access to toilets, and hand washing using soap.
- The diet should contain food that is easily digestible and one should minimize greasy and spicy food.
- Clinicians should understand the signs and symptoms associated with ascariasis in order to take timely action to prevent it.

Enterobiasis (Nao Chong Bing 蛲虫病)

Enterobiasis, or pinworm infection, is a common human intestinal parasitic disease manifested with itching in the anal area, accompanied with anxiety, restless sleep, even pinworms in the stools. It was called line worm in ancient times since it is very thin like a line. The appearance and location of pinworms was mentioned as one of the nine kinds of parasites by *Zhu Bing Yuan Hou Lun* (General Treatise on the Causes and Symptoms of diseases) 610, It states "pinworms are very thin and small just like the small bug of a vegetable., it lives in the rectum." Pinworm of *Sheng Ji Zhong Lu* (The Complete Record of Holy Benevolence) 1111 points out that: "anal itching is due to the pinworm biting there." It describes this as the main manifestation of enterobiasis. Pinworm infections occur worldwide, and are particularly common in children from 4 to 6 years old. Pinworms are usually considered a nuisance rather than a serious disease. Elimination of the parasite from a family group or an institution can be complicated—either due to an incomplete cure or reinfection.

Etiology and Pathology

The main cause of pinworm infection occurs by eating food or drink contaminated with pinworm eggs. Female pinworms lay eggs in the anus during the night, which stimulates itching. The eggs are readily transmitted from their initial deposit near the anus to the fingernails, hands, night-clothing and bed linen. From here, eggs are further transmitted to food, water, furniture, toys, bathroom fixtures and other objects. When children suck their fingers or eat food with their hands, the eggs will enter the stomach and intestine, then hatch in the intestine. When the pinworms emerge from the anus, it causes severe anal itching. If there are a large number of pinworms in the intestine, it will cause spleen and stomach dysfunction and generate damp heat. The pinworm also consumes qi and blood, resulting in poor appetite, loose stool, abdominal pain, emaciation, dull complexion, and fatigue.

Diagnosis

Diagnostic Guidelines

Mild manifestations are anal itching that is worse during the night. Severe cases will have intense itching or erosion around the anus affecting the perineum, accompanied with anxiety, restlessness, poor appetite, nausea, vomiting, abdominal pain, loose stool, or bed wetting. There may be eggs or pinworms in the feces, or in the anus.

Differential Diagnosis

Clinicians must differentiate between pinworm infection and anal eczema. Anal eczema also has anal itching, but the itching happens during the day and night. There will be a local rash and no pinworm eggs are found in the anus.

Diagnostic Notes

- Inquire if there is restlessness, anal itching, or nocturia.
- Observe if there are rashes, or erosion of the skin around the anus. Observe if there are pinworms emerging from the anus at night.
- Repeatedly check the stool and try to find pinworm eggs.

Pattern Differentiation

Guidelines of Differentiation

First determine the severity of case. If there is only anal itching and no other symptoms, it is a mild case. If there is severe itching or erosion around the anus affecting the perineum, accompanied with anxiety, restless, poor appetite, nausea, vomiting, abdominal pain, loose stool, or bed wetting, it is a severe case.

Next, determine any distal damage. Frequent, urgent, and painful urination with abdominal pain, it possibly indicates Lin syndrome, abnormal vaginal discharge, and intestinal carbuncle are distal damages from enterobiasis.

Therapeutic principle

The basic principle is to kill the pinworms. If there is vacuity of the spleen and stomach, we may also strengthen the spleen and stomach. If reinfection can be controlled, the treatment with herbal formula or drugs is not necessary.

Manifestations

Mild cases only show anal itching and restlessness. Severe cases, in addition to the itching, may be accompanied by anxiety, restlessness, poor appetite, nausea, vomiting, abdominal pain, loose stool, bed wetting, thin white or thin yellow tongue coating and a thin pulse.

Treatment principle Kill the pinworm, stop itching, and topical therapy.

Formula

Chu Chong Fen (Expel worms powder).

In the formula, the ratio of Shi Jun Zi (Fructus Quisqualis) and Da Huang (Radix et Rhizoma Rhei) is 8:1. Oral dosage is (year age+ 1) × 0.3g before meals, 3 times per day. 7~10 days is one course of treatment. 1~2 course for the case. Decoct Bai Bu 30g and get 30ml of liquid for enema before going to bed, every night for 10 days. Shi Jun Zi (Fructus Quisqualis) kills pinworms. Da Huang expels worms. Bai Bu (Radix Stemonae) kills worms and stops itching. If there is poor appetite, nausea, vomiting, abdominal pain, loose stool, add Shen Ling Bai Zhu San (Ginseng, Poria, and Atractylodes Macrocephala Powder).

Other therapy

- Hua Chong Wan (Resolve Worm Pills) Take orally 5g, TID. It is used for enterobiasis due to damp-heat with slow bowel movement.

- Vegetable oil is used topically by rubbing into the folds of the anus 1x/day before sleep.
- Decoct Bai Bu (Radix Stemonae) 20g and She Chuang Zi (Fructus Cnidii Monnieri) 15g. Wash the anus with this herbal decoction 1x/day.

Prevention and care

- Wash hands with soap and warm water after using the toilet, changing diapers, and before handling food
- In order to stop the spread of pinworms and possible re-infection, people who are infected should bathe every morning to help remove a large amount of the eggs on the skin.
- Infected people should not bathe with others during the time they are infected.
- They should also cut their fingernails regularly, and avoid biting the nails and scratching around the anus. Frequent changing of underclothes and bed linens first thing in the morning is a great way to prevent possible transmission of eggs into the environment and reduce the risk of re-infection.

Other Disorders
(Qi Ta Ji Bing 其它疾病)

The disorders in this chapter are related to the internal zang fu organs. This includes new diseases of Western pediatrics, such as rickets, purpura, and Kawasaki's disease. These disorders are due to functional disorders or physical damage to the zang f u. Therefore, it is necessary to understand the foundation of Western medicine and combine TCM theory for TCM practitioners. Although children's eczema is a skin disorder, it is very common in clinic. It is introduced in this chapter.

Night Crying (Ye Ti 夜 啼)

Night crying is when the baby is crying and restless during the night and may even cry all night, but the child does not cry during the day. It was noted in *Lu Xin Jin* (Classics of Skull and Fontanelle) and *Zhu Bing Yuan Hou Lun* (General Treatise on the Causes and Symptoms of diseases) 610 that "The night crying of children is due to cold in the zang fu organs."

The incidence of night crying is higher in newborn infants. Mostly the prognosis is good, but if it lasts for a long period, it may also affect normal growth and development of children.

The crying might result from hunger, wet diaper, fever, sores, abdominal pain and trauma, in which case refer to the appropriate chapters.

Etiology and pathology

Night crying is caused by cold in the spleen, heat in the heart and fear.

Cold with spleen vacuity Pregnant women who have a cold constitution, or eat too much cold food, will transfer interior cold into the spleen of infants. The cold invades infants when they take a bath or receive improper care. All of them may lead to cold stagnation in the spleen, resulting in night crying due to abdominal pain.

Heat accumulates in the heart The Yang of children tends to be replete. If a pregnant woman has a heat-type constitution, or eats too much spicy, dry and baked food, it results in interior heat accumulating in the heart of the infant. The heat pathogen is yang, and the heart in five phases is fire, two of the yang meet together, yang can't go into the inside of the body(yin) during the night, therefore, night crying occurs due to the heart-mind being disturbed by heat.

Sudden fear The heart stores the mind *Shen* (spirit), the liver stores the Hun (ethereal-soul), the lung stores the Po (corporeal-soul). If the zang fu organs are harmonized, the mind will be serene, Hun and Po will be peaceful, and therefore, children can calmly fall asleep. Children's brain and nervous systems haven't developed. If there is a sudden loud noise or strange noise, the children become fearful, Qi is disordered, and disturbs the heart mind, the Hun and Po are upset, resulting in night crying.

Diagnosis

Diagnostic Guidelines

- Crying every night, restless, but the child looks healthy and falls asleep during day. Not many abnormal signs on physical exam.
- There are no other disorders, such as fever, cough, asthma, food stagnation diarrhea, ulcers in mouth, ear infection and intussusception.

Differential Diagnosis

The night crying has to be differentiated from the disorders that may cause crying, such as fever, cough, asthma, food stagnation diarrhea, ulcers in mouth, ear infection, rickets and intussusception.

Diagnostic notes

- The age of children, when and how long the children cry should be inquired.
- The characteristics of the crying, state of spirit when the children cry and abdominal condition should be carefully observed and palpated.
- Note if it is due to hunger, thirst, cold and heat, wet diaper, tight clothing, or turning off the light.

Pattern Differentiation

Differentiation guidelines

- Differentiate between weeping and crying. If there is only weeping with sound but without tears, it is abdominal pain due to Qi stagnation. If there is crying with sound and tears, it is anxiety or fear.
- Differentiating between cold, heat and fear. If the crying sound is weak, a pale complexion, cold extremities, curled sleep, the abdomen likes to be pressed, pale tongue and white coating, it is due to cold. If the crying sound is loud, reddish face, hot body, anxiety, red tongue and yellow coating, it is heat. If the child suddenly cries, green face, expression of fear, crying is intermittent, it is fear.

Therapeutic Principle

The main principle is warming the spleen, clearing heart and calming fear.

Patterns and treatment

Cold invading due to the spleen vacuity

Manifestations

Night crying, weak crying, pale complexion, cold extremities, loose stool, profuse urine, curled sleep, the abdomen likes to be pressed, pale tongue and white coating, pale index vein.

Treatment Principle Warm the spleen and expel cold, regulate qi and stop pain.

Formula

Yun Qi San(Harmony Qi Powder)
   In the formula, Sha Ren (Radix Adenphorae seu Gleniae), Chen Pi (Pericarpium Citri Reticulatae), Mu Xiang (radix Aucklandiae Lappae) regulates qi and stop pain. Jie Geng (Radix Platycodi Grandifori) regulates qi, open chest, Pao Jiang (Quick-fried Rhisoma Zingberis Officinalis) and Zhi Gan Cao (honey-fried Radix Glycyrrhizae Uralensis) warm the middle and relax spasm. If the cold is severe, Wu Yao San (Linderae Powder) is modified.

Heat accumulating in heart channel

Manifestations

Night crying that is loud, worse after seeing the light, reddish face and lips, hot body, anxiety, yellow urine and constipation, red tongue and yellow coating purple and stagnated index vein.

Treatment Principle Clear heart, relieve anxiety and stop cry.

Formula

Xie Xin Dao Chi San (Drain the Heart and Guid Out the Red Decoction).

In the formula, Huang Lian (rhizoma coptidis) and Sheng Di Huang (Radix Rehmanniae Glutinosae) clear the heart and relieve anxiety. Dan Zhu Ye (Herba loptatheri gracilis), Gan Cao (Radix Glycyrrhizae Uralensis). add Da Huang (Radix et Rhizoma Rhei) purges the Fu organs. If there is severe anxiety, add Yuan Zhi (Radix Polygalae Tenuifoliae), Bai Zi Ren (Semen biotae orientalis). If the heat is sever in the heart, add Lian Qiao (Fructus forsythiae suspensae) and Zhi Zi (Fructus Gardeniae Jasminoidis).

Sudden fear

Manifestations

Sudden cry that is very loud, the complexion is suddenly purple, reddish and pale, scared complexion, or jerky, purple index vein.

Treatment principle Anchor the fear and calm the mind.

Formula

Zhu Sha An Shen Wan (Cinnabar Pill to Calm the Spirit)
    In the formula, Zhu Sha (Cinnabar) anchors fear, but it is toxic, Yuan Zhi (Radix Polygalae Tenuifoliae) and Gou Teng (Ramulus Cum Uncis Uncariae) replace it. Huang Lian (Rhizoma Coptidis) clears heat and relieves anxiety. Dang Gui (Radix Angelicae Sinensis) and Sheng Di Huang (Radix Rehmanniae Glutinosae) nourish blood and calm the mind.

Other therapy

Patent herbs

- Hu Po Bao Long Wan (Amber Hold Dragon Pill) ½ pill per time, 3 times per day. It is used for sudden fear.
- Jin Huang Bao Long Wan Golden Hold Dragon Pill) ½ pill per time, 3 times per day. It is used for heat accumulating in the heart.

Acupuncture

PC9, LI4, PC6, Du20. If the crying is due to heat, add PC7, and Lu11. If there is fear, add Ht7 and Liv2. Purging and not retaining needles. Bleeding PC9. Moxa Ren 8 for night crying due to cold.

Tuina

Push San Guan (three gates), reduce Six Fu, clear heart and divide Yin and Yang. If it is due to cold, add push spleen and kneading at St36. If it is due to heat, add kneading general tendons and kneading of Liv2. If it is due to fear, add kneading on Ht7 and St41.

Topical therapy

- Heat Dan Dou Chi (Semen Sojae Praeparatum) 10g, sliced Sheng Jiang (Rhizoma Zingiberis Recens) 6g, sliced Cong Bai (Bulbus Allii Fistulosi) 6g and salt 10g, then wrap them together, put it on the umbilicus. It is used for cold with spleen vacuity.
- Heat the Ai Ye (Folium Artemisiae Argyi) 30g Gan Jiang(Rhizoma Zingiberis) 30g, and wrap them, put it on the lower abdomen. It is used for cold with spleen vacuity.

Prevention and care

- Avoid eating spicy, hot and cold foods during pregnancy.
- Keep the environment quiet and harmonized.
- Keep newborns warm without overheating.
- Educate children about good sleep habits.

Profuse Sweating (Han Zheng 汗证)

If there is profuse sweating all over the body or local areas at rest, it is a sweating syndrome. These were named as profuse sweating, leaking sweating and sleep sweating in the *Huang Di Nei Jing*. It was divided as two pattern in the *Zhu Bing Yuan Huo Lun* (General

Treatise on the Causes and symptoms of diseases, children's syndromes) 610 stated "since the qi and blood of children are not sufficient and their skin striae is porous, or if their clothing is too thick or the covers are too warm, it will generate heat in the zang fu, steam in the striae, and body fluid leaks outside, which results in sweating". "The night sweating is manifested with sweat during sleep. The qi of yin and yang of children is tender, their striae tends to open. Since the Yin and Yang are crossing during night, if the covering is too hot, the body fluid leaks, resulting in sweating. " *Xiao Er Yao Zheng Zhi Jue* (Key to Differentiation and Treatment of Disease of Children) 1119 also discusses the syndromes of profuse sweating, night sweating and Taiyang vacuity sweating, which are treated by formulas, such as Zhi Han San (Stop sweat powder) and Xiang Gua San (Fragrant melon Powder). Perspiration is the body fluid which is evaporated by yang and regulated by Wei Qi, and sent to the skin through the pores. Sweating is the physical activity of the crossing of yin and yang, Ying and Wei, regulating the body temperature, moistening the muscles and skin, and expelling waste from the body. The physical functions of children are vigorous, and their striae are not so airtight, therefore, children have more sweating than adults. If children have increased sweating because they are over dressed in hot weather, or they are fed too fast, or they are too active, but no other abnormal manifestations, they are still considered as healthy. There are two patterns of sweating syndromes, which are spontaneous sweating and night sweating. The sweating occurs during sleep and stops when awake, it is night sweating, it is likely due to yin vacuity. When sweating occurs during day without movement, it is spontaneous sweating, it is likely due to Yang Qi vacuity. In clinic, night sweating and spontaneous sweating often occur in the same child. The sweating also may occur in other diseases or syndromes, such as children with febrile warm disease, rickets, or yang collapse. If that is the case, physicians have to consider a combination of diseases or syndromes for treatment.

Etiology and pathology

The profuse sweating syndrome is caused by weakened exterior Qi, vacuity of Qi and Yin and, heat accumulation in the heart and spleen.

Weakened exterior qi "Spontaneous sweating is related to Yang vacuity, Wei Qi is weak so that striae are not airtight, the body fluid leaks out through striae resulting in spontaneous sweating."(Jing Yue Chuan Shu).

Vacuity of qi and yin The constitutions of children are pure Yang, they suffer heat syndromes easily. If the heat syndromes occurs frequently or long term, Qi and Yin are going to be damaged, the weak Qi and Yin become disordered and the opening and closing function of the striae fails, resulting in profuse sweating.

Heat accumulation of the heart and spleen If the care or diet for children disagrees with them, it may cause heat accumulation of the heart and spleen, or the dampness generated from the spleen stagnates and turns to damp heat over a long term, excessive Yang leads to imbalance of Yin and Yang, and spontaneous sweating.

Diagnosis

Diagnostic Guidelines

- Consider if the sweating is local or all over the body, whether it occurs during night or without exertion, but exclude over dressing, or very hot weather
- Profuse sweating might be spontaneous with night sweating occurring with the same patient, which often wet their clothes and pillows.

Diagnostic Notes

- Note the sweating due to a physiological condition.
- Note the children's age, history of feeding, growth and development. Inquire whether the children have had

long-term fever, cough, weight loss, fatigue and poor appetite. Palpate if there is any superficial lymph nodes.

- Note history of vaccinations and exposure to infectious diseases. Carefully observe the throat, rash, etc., in order to clarify whether there are other disease mechanisms present.
- Necessarily combine with general blood test, erythrocyte sedimentation rate, anti-"O", serum calcium and phosphorus, tuberculin test, X-ray and other examinations to make sure the sweating is not secondary from other diseases.

Pattern Differentiation

Differentiation guidelines

Children often have spontaneous and night sweating concurrently, repletion and vacuity are the main criteria evaluated in profuse sweating in clinic. If there is sweating all over the body, susceptibility to cold, poor appetite, fatigue, thin pulse, or after chronic illness, it is likely due to vacuity. If the sweating is more at the head or extremities, strong constitution, constipation, scanty urine, it is likely repletion.

Therapeutic principle

The main principle is to harmonize Yin and Yang and try to balance the yin and yang.

Patterns and treatment

Weakened exterior qi

Manifestations

More spontaneous sweating than night sweating, all over the body, worse when active, pale complexion, poor appetite, susceptibility to cold, pale tongue with less coating, thin and weak pulse.

Treatment Principle Supplement qi, stabilize the exterior and stop sweating

Formula

Yu Ping Feng San (Jade Windscreen Powder) and Mu Li (Concha Ostreae Powder)

In the formula, Huang Qi (Radix Astragali Membranaceus) and Mu Li (Concha Ostreae) supplement Qi and stabilize the exterior, Bai Zhu (Rhizoma Atractylodis) strengthens the spleen and Fang Feng (Redix Ledebouriella Divaricatae) goes to the exterior to expel wind.

Vacuity of qi and yin

Manifestations

Often occurs after febrile or chronic disease, more night sweating than spontaneous sweating, which is all over the body, fatigue, anxiety and insomnia, also accompanied lower grade fever, hot sensation of hands and feet, thirsty, pale tongue with less coating or peeled coating, thin and weak pulse.

Treatment Principle Supplement qi and nourish yin.

Formula

Sheng Mai San (Generate Pulse Powder).

In the formula, Ren Shen (Radix Ginseng) and Mai Men Dong (Tuber Ophiopogonis Japonici) supplement Qi and nourish Yin, Wu Wei Zi (Fructus Schisandrae Chunensis) astringes the lung, generates body fluids and stops sweating. If qi vacuity is severe, also add Huang Qi (Radix Astragali Membranaceus) for strengthening the defensive Qi. If there is lower grade fever, add Huang Bai (Cotex Phellodendri), Zhi mu (Rhizome Anemarrhenae), Xuan Shen (Radix scrophulariae Ningpoensis) and Sheng Di Huang (Uncooked Radix Rehmanniae) to nourish Yin and sedate fire. If there is severe sweating, add Fu Xiao Mai (Semen Tritici Aestivi

Levis), Long Gu (Os Draconis) and Mu Li (Concha Ostreae) to stop sweating. If there is anxiety and insomnia, add Ye Jiao Teng (Caulis Polygoni Multiflori), Suan Zao Ren (Semen Zizyphi Spinosae) to calm spirit.

Heat accumulation of the heart and spleen

Manifestations

Spontaneous or night sweating, which is yellow, strong smell and more at the head and extremities, bad breath, sores on the tongue, thirst and anxiety, scanty urine and constipation, red tongue with yellow and greasy coating, slippery and rapid pulse.

Treatment Principle Clear the heart, purge spleen and eliminate dampness.

Formula

Xie Huang San (Purge Yellow Powder) and Dao Chi San (Guide Red Powder).

In the formula, Shi Gao (Gypsum) and Zhi Zi (Fructus Gardeniae Jasminoidis) clear heat of the spleen and stomach. Fang Feng (Redix Ledebouriella Divaricatae) expels evils inside of the body, Huo Xiang (Herba Agastaches Seu Pogostemi) harmonizes the middle and eliminates dampness. Sheng Di Huang (Radix Rehmanniae Glutinosae) clears heat and cools blood. Zhu Ye (Bamboo Leaf) and Gan Cao (Radix Glycyrrhizae Uralensis) clear heart and purge heat.

Other Therapy

- Yu Ping Feng Jiaonang (Jade Windscreen Capsule) taken orally 1 capsule, twice a day. It is used for weakened exterior qi.
- Shen Mai Yin Koufuye (Generate Pulse Liquid) taken orally 1 bottle, twice a day. It is used for vacuity of Qi and Yin.

313

Prevention and Care

- Do more outdoor activities to enhance the physical constitution.
- Rational feeding, add the complementary food for the child in time.
- Avoid eating spicy fragrant, dry and greasy foods.
- The patient who has profuse sweating should drink more water, eat food that is easily digested and nutritious.

Five retardations and Five Flabbinesses (Wu Chi, Wu Ruan五迟、五软)

Five retardations are manifestations of growth tardiness or ability to stand, to walk and to speak, and of growth of the hair and the teeth. The five flabbinesses sluggish movement caused by underdevelopment in infants, is flabbiness of the neck, hands and feet, muscles and of the mouth. The five retardations and five flabbinesses can occur separately or together, but their pathologies are similar. These syndromes and their pathologies are recorded in *Zhu Bing Yuan Hou Lun* (General Treatise on the Causes and Symptoms of diseases) 610. *Xiao Er Yao Zheng Zhi Jue* (Key to Differentiation and Treatment of Disease of Children) 1119 also discusses the syndromes of five retardations and five flabbinesses, which relates to acquired and innate factors, but if it is due to congenital factors, the progress is poor.

Etiology and pathology

The syndrome may be caused by congenital vacuity, acquired dystrophy, birth trauma, and side effects of medications. The kidneys are the root of the innate, they stores essence and take charge of the bones and generate marrow. If the weak essence of the parents fails to nourish the fetus, it affects the fetus' essence insufficiently, resulting in weak bones. The spleen is responsible for the normality of muscles, activity of the extremities and postnatal growth of the human body. If the spleen and stomach are damaged by incorrect care and feeding, it might weaken the nutrition from the spleen and stomach, and fail to nourish the muscles; therefore the muscles and extremities become weak. The pathology of the five retardations and five flabbinesses are focused on the spleen and kidney.

Vacuity of liver and kidney If there is an insufficiency of spleen and kidney Qi, the liver blood is weak and fails to nourish the tendons and bones, resulting in weak bones and tendons and tardiness of the ability to stand, to walk with flabbiness of neck, hands and feet.

Vacuity of heart and spleen If children suffer vacuity of the spleen and kidney, their Qi and blood are insufficiently produced, which results in the failure to nourish the heart and hair, therefore, the growth and tardiness of the ability to speak, of hair growth and the teeth occurs, and is accompanied with flabbiness of the muscles and mouth.

Diagnosis

Diagnostic Guidelines

- If a child who is two or three years old is not able to stand and walk, it is considered to be a case of delayed development. In addition there is very little or no hair after birth, minimal or slight hair growth is another symptom of delayed development. Little or no growth of teeth is another symptom. If they are unable to speak after two years old, it may be accompanied with low intelligence. The neck may be too weak and soft to be able to support the head, and the head droops down, this is neck flabbiness. If the muscles of the mouth are too weak to chew food and droops saliva, it is mouth flabbiness; If there is weakness of the hands, and arms to grasp and rise up, it is hand flabbiness. If the muscles of the legs are too weak to support the body it is leg flabbiness; soft and weak muscles are considered as muscle flabbiness.

- There is a history of incorrect therapy during pregnancy, birth trauma, asphyxia, premature delivery, jaundice of newborn, and incorrect nursing.

Differential Diagnosis

Rickets It occurs under 2 years of age, mostly due to acquired factors. Although there can be the manifestations of five delay and five flabbiness, it is mild, which may accompanied by profuse sweating and easily scared. It also easily affects bones and muscles, but no dementia. The prognosis of rickets usually is good and can be completely recovered.

Hydrocephalus It may have manifestations of five delay and five flabbiness, but the patient also has the following signs of separated sutures of skull, enlargement of the head, mental disability, drooped head and eyes that appear to gaze downward.

Diagnostic Notes

- Inquire about the child's age, history of delivery, development, nursing and family.
- Carefully observe the hair, teeth, complexion, and posture of standing and walking, and spirit as well.
- Necessarily check blood test, CT or DNA.

Pattern Differentiation

Differentiation guidelines

- Differentiate the severity of the case. If there is only one or two of manifestations of the five delay and five flabbiness, with normal intelligence, it is a mild syndrome. If there are all of the manifestations of five delay and five flabbiness, it is a severe syndrome.

- Differentiate the Zang Fu syndrome: The locations of five delay and five flabbiness focus on the spleen and kidney. If the manifestations are tardiness of ability to stand, to walk, to grow teeth and flabbiness of the neck, hands and feet, it is related to vacuity of liver, spleen and kidney. If there is tardiness of the ability to grow hair and to speak, and flabbiness of muscles and of mouth, and mental retardation, it is vacuity of heart, spleen and kidney.

Therapeutic Principle

Focus on supplementing liver and kidney, strengthening spleen and nourishing heart. However, the effects are not going to happen in the short-term only with internal treatment, it requires not only comprehensive and long-term therapy, therapy should also include functional exercises, mental training and rehabilitation.

Patterns and Treatment

Vacuity of liver and kidney

Manifestations

Late ability to stand, stand and set, late growth teeth than of children of the same age. Flabby neck and muscles, shaking hands and feet, pale tongue with thin coating, deep and weak pulse.

Treatment Principle Nourish kidney and generate liver, strengthen essence and supplement marrow.

Formula

Liu Wei Di Huang Wan (Six-ingredient pill with Rehmannia).
In the formula, Shu Di Huang (Radix Rehmanniae Glutinosae Conquitae) and Shan Zhu Yu (Fructus Corni Officinalis) nourish the kidney and generate liver. Shan Yao (Radix Dioscoreae Oppositae)

and Fu Ling (Sclerotium Poria Cocos) strengthen spleen and fill essence. Ze xie (Rhizoma Alismatis Orientalis) and Mu Dan Pi (Cortex Moutan Radicis) eliminates dampness and clears the liver. Add Gui Ban (Turtle Shell) to strengthen bones and tendons. if there are flabby muscles, add Dang Shen (Radix Codonopsitis Pilosulae), Bai Zhu (Rhizoma Atractylodis) and Huang Qi (Radix Astragali Membranaceus) If there are shaking hands and feet, add Tian Ma (Rhizoma Gastrodiae Elatae) and Gou Teng (Ramulus Cum Uncis Uncariae). If there is mental retardation, add Shi Chang Pu (Rhizoma Acori Graminei), Yuan Zhi(Radix Polygalae Tenuifoliae).

Vacuity of heart and spleen

Manifestations

Lower intelligence, pale complexion, slow speech, flaccidity of muscles, slow walking and poor appetite, drooling, outstretched tongue, pale tongue with less coating, thin and weak pulse.

Treatment principle Nourish heart and strengthen spleen.

Formula

Tiao Yuan San (Regulate Yuan Powder) and Chang Pu Wan (Acori Graminei Pills).

In the formula, Ren Shen (Radix Ginseng), Huang Qi (Radix Astragali Membranaceus), Fu Ling (Sclerotium Poria cocos) and Bai Zhu (Rhizoma Atractylodis) strengthen spleen and supplement qi. Dang Gui (Radix Angelicae Sinesis), Shu Di Huang (Radix Rehmanniae Glutinosae Conquitae), Chuan Xiong (Radix Lgustici Chuanxiong) nourish Yin and generate blood. Shi Chang Pu (Rhizoma Acori Graminei), Yuan Zhi (Radix polygalae tenuifoliae) nourish the heart and open orifice. If there is thin hair, add He Shou Wu (Radix Polygoni Multiflori) and Fleshy Stem of Broomrape. If there is poor appetite, add Mu Gua (Chaenomeles Lagenaria) and Huo Xiang (Herba Agastaches Seu Pogostemi).

Other Therapy

Tuina

- Pushing, kneading and rolling the head, body and acupuncture points, which can activate blood and unblock channels, nourish tendons and muscles, relax meridians, rectify the functional movement. Tuina 1~2 times per day, total 10-15 times as a course of therapy.
- For Head and face: Patients sitting. Kneading forwards and backwards on GB1, St3,St4, GB20, Du15, Du20 and UB10. 5~6 times per day.
- For Neck and upper Extremities: Patient sitting. Knead from UB10 to DU14 and GB21. Push and knead from shoulders, triceps and biceps section to elbows. 5-6 times per day.
- For Lower Back and Lower Extremities: Prone position. Push and knead from lower back to sacral, hip, and along exterior of legs to heel. Press the related points that are UB23, UB21, Liv3, GB30,UB37, UB40 and UB57.

Moxibustion

UB15, UB21, UB23 and related regular acupuncture points. Once per day, 10 times as a course of treatment. Avoid burning their skin, since the kids' skin is tender.

Acupuncture

Choose from these points, such as LI14, LI11, SJ5, LI4, GB30, St36, GB34, UB57 and Sp6. Do not retain needles. If there is mental retardation, add Du20, GB20, Ht7 and Du15. Retain the needles for 15~20 minutes. Once every other day. One month as a course of treatment.

Ear acupuncture

Heart, liver, kidney, stomach, brain stem, adrenal gland. Retain 15-20 minutes, once every other day. 15 times treatment as a course.

Prevention and care

- Pay attention to the maternal health and prevent infection and side effects of medication; Avoid premature birth, birth trauma and dytsocia; prevent pneumonia of newborn and sclerodema neonatorum.
- Reasonable feeding and nutrition, actively prevent and treat various acute and chronic diseases.
- Do exercises for the limb function and train linguistic intelligence.

Vitamin D deficiency Rickets
(Wei Sheng Shu D Que Fa Xing Gou
Lou Bing 维生素缺乏性佝偻病)

Vitamin D deficiency causes rickets, a name in Western medicine, and it is a disorder of defective mineralization of bones due to the deficiency or impaired metabolism of vitamin D and phosphorus, manifested with anxiety, night crying, profuse sweating, muscle weakness, cranial deformity, square headed-ness, delayed fontanel closure, rosary beads, pigeon chest, bowed legs. Vitamin D deficiency rickets is among the most frequent childhood diseases in many developing countries. It often occurs under 2 years childhood and it is of higher incidence in the north more than in the south. Prognosis is generally good, if rickets is not corrected while the child is still growing, skeletal deformities and short stature may be permanent. If it is corrected while the child is young, skeletal deformities often improve or disappear with time. It was discussed as five delay, five flabbiness, night crying, pigeon chest and tortoise back. The *Zhu Bing Yuan Hou Lun* (General Treatise on the Causes and Symptoms of diseases) 610 suggests a prevention for them is "more exposure to sunlight."

Etiology and Pathology

This is a disorder caused by vacuity of spleen and kidney due to congenital insufficiency, incorrect feeding and care.

Congenital insufficiency The following are causes that lead to congenital insufficiency, such as the mother who is incorrectly nursing during pregnancy, insufficient sunlight, malnutrition, or other chronic diseases, all of them will affect the fetal development, resulting in congenital weakness and insufficiency of kidney.

Incorrect care after birth weak qi and blood occurs due to the child being fed insufficient breast milk or formula, which fails to nourish Zang and Fu, and both spleen and kidney becoming injured, then illness occurs.

Children who have little outdoor activities, or haven't been exposed to sunlight for long periods or they are born in cold regions without enough sunlight, will have insufficient skeletal growth and they will not be strong; just like grasses and flowers without sunlight won't grow inside the house. The main causes are insufficient spleen and kidneys due to congenital insufficiency and incorrect care after birth. Kidney vacuity fails to nourish bones, leading to slow growth and development, Asymmetrical or odd-shaped skull, pigeon chest and spinal deformities. The spleen fails to generate qi and blood so that can't nourish muscles and skin and hair, resulting in weak muscles, thin and sparse hair, also susceptibility to cold. Hyperascendent liver yang due to liver blood vacuity, results in anxiety and night crying. The tendon are not properly nourished, therefore standing and walking are weak. The heart qi is damaged causing lower intelligence and tardiness in the ability to speak.

Diagnosis

Diagnostic Guidelines

Early stage manifestations

Profuse sweating, anxiety, restlessness, scared and crying the during night, also may have delayed formation of teeth and fontanel closure, or baldness.

Agitated stage

The above symptoms including bone tenderness soft skull, delayed fontanel closure widening of the wrists, bowed legs, knock-knees, kyphoscoliosis or lumbar lordosis. This often occurs in infants three months to 2 years old or children who have inadequate outdoor activities. Inadequate amounts of complementary foods rich in vitamin D early in life.

Rickets may be diagnosed with the help of:

- Serum calcium may show low levels of calcium, serum phosphorus may be low, and serum alkaline phosphatase may be high from bones or changes in the shape or structure of the bones. This can show enlarged limbs and joints.
- An X-ray or radiograph shows bowed legs and a deformed chest, skull also occur "square headed" appearance.

Differential Diagnosis

- *Jie Lu (hydrocephalus)* It may have manifestations of five delay and five flabbiness, but the patient also has the following characteristics of separated skull sutures, enlargement of the head, mental disability, drooped head and eyes that appear to gaze downward
- This disease still needs to be differentiated from congenital hypothyroidism, malnutrition of cartilage and various types of rickets due to other disorders.

Diagnostic Notes

- Note the child's age, the onset of the season, ask in detail about the history of feeding, growth and outdoor activities.
- Notice if the child has irritability, night crying, a vacant look, loss of appetite, sweating, frequent sickness and constant colds or other medical history.

- Observe the hair, head, fontanel, chest, spine and limbs and so on.
- Do the following tests if necessary: serum calcium, phosphorus, alkaline phosphatase and X-ray examination.

Pattern Differentiation

Differentiation guidelines

Differentiate stages:

The early stage

Aanxiety, profuse sweating, baldness, night crying, no skeletal deformities

The agitated stage

In addition to the manifestations of the early stage, also shows skeletal deformities and sluggish activity.

The recovery stage

The manifestations disappear after being treated.

The sequelae stage

There are skeletal deformities after agitated stage.

Differentiate the zang and fu The manifestations of the early stage, such as soft muscles, poor appetite, loose feces, thin and sparse hair, susceptibility to cold, related to lung and spleen vacuity; The manifestations, such as anxiety, profuse sweating, baldness, night crying, skeletal deformities and sluggish activity, related to the heart, liver and kidney.

Differentiate between the mild and the severe If there is mild skull tenderness, square headed, rosary beads, delayed fontanel closure, it is a mild case. If there are typical skeletal deformities, such as rosary beads, widening of wrists, even pigeon chest, scoliosis, bowed legs and skeletal fractures it is a severe case.

Therapeutic Principle

Strengthen the spleen and generate qi, supplement kidney and generate essence. If it is at the early stage, strengthen spleen and supplement lung. strengthen spleen and calm liver, or supplement kidney and generate essence for severe case at the agitated stage. During the active stage, the main purpose is to prevent recurrence of deformity. Try to adopt comprehensive measures, including sunlight and reasonable diet to prevent complication.

Patterns and treatment

Qi vacuity of the lung and spleen

Manifestations

Loose muscles, pale complexion, poor appetite, profuse sweating, loose feces, restlessness, thin and sparse hair, susceptibility to cold, pale tongue with thin white coating, pale index vein, deep weak pulse.

Treatment principle Strengthen spleen and supplement lungs, generate qi and consolidate exterior.

Formula

Yu Ping Feng San (Jade Windscreen Powder) and Ren Shen Wu Wei Zi San (Ginseng and Schisandrae Powder)

In the formula, Huang Qi (Radix Astragali Membranaceus) supplements qi and consolidates the exterior. Wu Wei Zi (Fructus Schisandrae Chinensis), Bai Zhu (Rhizoma Atractylodis) and Fang Feng (Redix Ledebouriella Divaricatae), Fu Ling (Sclerotium Poria Cocos) and Ren Shen (Radix Ginseng) strengthen spleen, generate qi and supplement the lungs. Mai Men Dong (Tuber Ophiopogonis Japonici) and Wu Wei Zi (Fructus Schisandrae Chunensis) astringe the lungs, generate body fluids and stop sweating. Fang Feng (Redix Ledebouriella Divaricatae) goes to the exterior to expel wind. If there is profuse sweating, add Long Gu (Os Draconis) and Mu Li (Concha Ostreae) to stop sweating. If there is anxiety and insomnia, add Ye Jiao Teng (Caulis Polygoni Multiflori), Suan Zao Ren (Semen Zizyphi Spinosae) to calm the spirit. If there are loose feces, add Shan Yao (Radix Dioscoreae Oppositae) and Bai Bian Dou (Dolichos Lablab).

Spleen vacuity and liver hyperactivity

Manifestations

Pale complexion, profuse sweating, thin and sparse hair, poor appetite, no power to walk, night crying with fear, pale tongue with thin coating, pale index vein, thin and wiry pulse.

Treatment principle Supplement spleen and calm liver.

Formula

Yi Pi Zhen Jing San (Strengthen Spleen and Calm Frighten Powder)
    In the formula, Ren Shen (Radix Ginseng), Bai Zhu (Rhizoma Atractylodis), Fang Feng (Redix Ledebouriella Divaricatae) and Fu Ling (Sclerotium Poria Cocos) strengthen the spleen. Gou Teng (Ramulus Cum Uncis Uncariae) calms the liver and extinguishes wind. if there is profuse sweating, also add Wu Wei Zi (Fructus Schisandrae Chunensis), Long Gu (Os Draconis) and Mu Li (Concha Ostreae). If there is anxiety and insomnia, add Ye Jiao Teng (Caulis Polygoni Multiflori) and Suan Zao Ren (Semen Zizyphi Spinosae).

Vacuity of spleen and kidney

Manifestations

Widening of the wrists, pigeon chest, scoliosis, bowed legs and skeletal fractures, in addition to the manifestations of syndrome of spleen vacuity and liver hyperactivity, pale tongue with less coating, deep and weak pulse

Treatment Principle Supplement kidney and replenish essence

Formula

Bu Tian Da Zhao Wan (Supplement Heaven Major Product Pill)
    In the formula, Ren Shen (Radix Ginseng), Huang Qi (Radix Astragali Membranaceus) Bai Zhu (Rhizoma Atractylodis), Fu Ling (Sclerotium Poria Cocos) and Shan Yao (Radix Dioscoreae Oppositae) supplement spleen qi. Zi He Che (Dried Human Placenta), Lu Jiao (Cornu Cervii), Gui Ban (Plastrum Testudinis), Dang Gui (Radix Angelicae Sinensis), Gou Qi Zi (Fructus Lycii) and Shu Di Huang (Radix Rehmanniae Glutinosae Conquitae) supplement bones marrow and strengthen bones. Suan Zao Ren (Semen Zizyphi Spinosae) and Yuan Zhi (Radix Polygalae Tenuifoliae) nourish heart and calm the mind. If there is profuse sweating, also add Long Gu (Os Draconis) and Mu Li (Concha Ostreae) to stop sweating. If there is poor appetite, add Sha Ren (Radix Adenphorae Seu Gleniae), Chen Pi (Pericarpium Citri Reticulatae) to supplement and regulate the spleen and stomach. If there is a low IQ, add Shi Chang Pu (Rhizoma Acori Graminei) and Yu Jin Tuber Curcumae) to open the orifice and awaken the brain.

Other Therapy

Patent herbs

- Long Mu Zhuang Gu San (Os Draconis and Concha Ostreae Strengthen Powder) Taken orally 1 package, twice a day. It is used for qi vacuity of the lungs and spleen, and vacuity of the spleen and kidney as well.
- Yu Ping Feng Jiao Nang (Jade Windscreen Capsule) Taken orally 1 capsule, twice a day. It is used for weakened exterior qi.

- Liu Wei Di Huang Wan (Six-ingredient pill with Rehmannia) Taken orally 3-6g, three times per day. It is used for kidney and spleen vacuity.
- Vitamin D therapy You may refer to MD or nutritionist.

Prevention and Care

- Pregnant women should do more outdoor activities, get adequate exposure to sunlight and have good nutrition
- Recommend two months old infants exposure to sunlight more than average one hour a day
- Promote breastfeeding, add diets that are rich in vitamin D, calcium and phosphates early on

Purpura (Zi Dian 紫癜)

Purpura are the red or purple discolorations on the skin that is caused by bleeding underneath the skin, which includes two kinds of disorders. One is idiopathic thrombocytopenic purpura (ITP), and is purpura associated with a reduction in circulating blood platelets which can result from a variety of causes. The other common one is characterized by deposition of immune complexes. Two of the purpura are also often accompanied with bleeding at other locations, such as epistaxis, periodontal bleeding, blood in the stool and urine. Purpura most commonly affects school age children. Overall prognosis is good in most patients, but some of the cases can be longer in duration, and a few of them may have a poor prognosis due to intracranial hemorrhage. There was no purpura in ancient classics, but it related to bleeding syndromes and maculae (Ban) toxin. The *Zhu Bing Yuan Hou Lun* (General Treatise on the Causes and Symptoms of diseases) 610 on maculae states maculae are due to "heat with toxin accumulating in the stomach and the heat toxin showing in the muscles."

Etiology and Pathology

This disorder is most commonly caused by heat that creates chaotic movement of hot blood, vacuity that fails to control the blood inside the vessels, or when yin can't astringe blood inside the vessels.

Wind heat injuring vessels The six evils tends to turn to heat because of the pure yang constitution of children. If the exterior pathogens invade the body, then turn to heat and injures vessels, blood leaks out of the vessels, stays under skin, resulting in purpura. If the blood that leaks out from vessels stays in stomach and intestine, it may cause abdominal pain and bleeding in the feces. If wind-heat with dampness floods downwards, and burns the vessels of the urinary bladder, it may lead to hematuria. If it floods to the joints, there will be swollen and painful joints.

Chaotic movement due to hot blood Exterior evils invading body from the Wei level to qi, and even Ying and blood. When the heat enters the Ying and blood level, it increases the blood to move recklessly and it leaves its normal pathways, and leaks into the skin, resulting in purpura. In the upper part of the body, this manifests as nosebleed and gums bleeding. In the middle of the stomach and intestines, it presents as vomiting of blood and blood in the stool. in the lower urinary bladder, as hematuria. If there is too much blood loss or repeated bleeding, it may cause exhaustion of qi and blood.

Loss of blood retention due to qi vacuity If there is spleen vacuity due to incorrect diet, or chronic disorders, the spleen qi fails to control blood in its normal pathways, and the bleeding occurs under skin. This manifests as purpura, nosebleed and bleeding gums.

Yin vacuity of liver and kidney Congenital vacuity or chronic disorders that leads to yin vacuity of the liver and kidney, the vacuous heat forces blood to move recklessly and leave its pathways, resulting in purpura and bleeding.

In summary, the purpura results from heat or vacuity. If it is due to heat, mostly focus on treating the lungs and stomach, also treat liver and kidney. If vacuity is predominant, mostly treat spleen and heart, also treat liver and kidney. Since the blood is under the skin, it becomes blood stasis, invigorating blood stasis is also necessary.

Diagnosis

Diagnostic Guidelines

Manifestations of allergic purpura

The purpura typically appears on the legs and buttocks, but may also be seen on the arms, face and trunk. The abdominal pain is colicky in character, and may be accompanied by nausea, vomiting, constipation or diarrhea. There may be blood or mucus in the stools and urine. The joints involved tend to be the ankles, knees and elbows. Before it occurs, the patients have a history of infection (bacterial, virus, or parasites), or after taking medications, contaminated food, or exposure to allergens.

Laboratory exam: WBC and eosinophils may be slightly increased, normal platelet count, accelerated ESR, even RBC in urine.

Manifestations of idiopathic thrombocytopenic purpura

The spontaneous formation of bruises and tiny purpura, especially on the extremities, easily accompanied with bleeding from the nostrils, gums and excessive menstrual bleeding. If bleeding inside the brain occurs there may be unconsciousness. The patient's platelets count is extremely low.

Differentiation of Diagnose

Allergic purpura

It has to be differentiated from acute abdominal pain and rheumatoid arthritis if the allergic purpura shows abdominal pain or joints pain before it has purpura.

Idiopathic thrombocytopenic purpura

This should be distinguished from aplastic anemia, leukemia and other blood diseases.

Diagnostic Notes

Note the laboratory tests of blood that helps distinguish allergic purpura and idiopathic thrombocytopenic purpura.

- Note the patient's age, the shapes, color and locations of purpura.
- Note if there is any history of infection, allergies to medicine or food before the purpura occurs.
- Note check if there is fever, anemia, hepatomegaly, splenomegaly and lymphadenectasis.
- Check the abdomen, cardiovascular and nervous system, even bone marrow smear if necessary.

Pattern Differentiation

Differentiation guidelines

Differentiate between vacuity, repletion and stasis If it is at the early stage, the purpura are reddish and bright, it is mostly due to heat causing the blood move recklessly, which is a repletion syndrome. At the later and chronic stages, purpura occur repeatedly with pale color, and it is vacuity syndrome. If it also has abdominal pain, swollen and painful joints, purple tongue, it is accompanied with qi and blood stasis.

Differentiate between the mild and severe If the purpura are loose, no other bleeding or accompanying manifestations, it is a mild syndrome. If there are a lot of purpura, even bleeding with a pale complexion, cold extremities, and very deep and weak pulse, this is an exhaustion syndrome due to vacuity.

Integrate the differentiation syndrome and differentiation of diseases
According to the manifestations of diseases, the allergic purpura are
likely to show the symptoms of wind-heat injuring Luo meridians
and chaotic movement of hot blood. Idiopathic thrombocytopenic
purpura mostly shows syndromes of vacuity of the heart and
spleen, or vacuity of the spleen and kidney.

Therapeutic principle

Clear heat and expel wind, cool blood and stop bleeding is the
principle for heat in the blood. Supplement qi, stop bleeding,
nourish Yin and cool blood are for syndromes of blood vacuity
and Yin vacuity. Invigorate blood for the syndrome accompanied
with blood stasis.

Pattern and treatment

Wind-heat injuring the meridians

Manifestations

Reddish purpura that is of acute onset, maculae and rashes which
are located more on the lower legs and hips, accompanied with
itching, or occasionally with joint pain, abdominal pain, fecal and
urinary bleeding, red tongue with yellow coating, floating and
rapid pulse.

Treatment Principle Expel wind and clear heat, cool the blood
and stop bleeding.

Formula

Yin Qiao San (Honeysuckle and Forsythia Powder) modified.
  In the formula, Jing Jie (Herbs Seu Flos Schizonepetae
Tenuifoliae), Bo He (Herba Menthae Haplocalycis), Dan Dou
Chi (Semen Sojae Praeparatum), Jin Yin Hua (Flos Lonicerae
Japonicae) and Lian Qiao (Rhizoma Coptidis) clear heat and
toxin, expel wind and release the exterior. Add Mu Dan Pi (Cortex

Moutan Radicis), Chi Shao (Radix Paeoniae Rubra) and Sheng Di Huang (Radix Rehmanniae Glutinosae) to cool the blood. If there is skin itching, also add Fang Feng (Redix Ledebouriella Divaricatae) and Bai Xian Pi (Cortex Dictammi Dasycarpi). Add Mu Xiang (Radix Aucklandiae Lappae) and Yan Hu Suo (Corydalis Yanhusuo) for abdominal pain.

Chaotic movement due to hot blood

Manifestations

Acute onset, fever, anxiety, reddish or even deep reddish purpura over all body, strong odor, abdominal pain, constipation, accompanied with bleeding of nose, gums and feces, deep red tongue with yellow coating, full and rapid pulse.

Treatment Principle Clear heat and purge fire, cool and stop bleeding.

Formula

Hua Ban Tang (Transform Blotches Decoction) modified

In the formula: Zhi Zi (Fructus Gardeniae Jasminoidis), Shi Gao (Gypsum) and Zhi Mu (Rhizome Anemarrhenae) clear heat and purge fire. Fang Feng (Redix Ledebouriella Divaricatae) and Huo Xiang (Herba Agastaches Seu Pogostemi) expel wind and eliminates dampness. Sheng Di Huang (Radix Rehmanniae Glutinosae) and Xuan Shen (Radix Scrophulariae Ningpoensis) cool blood and stop bleeding. Add Huang Lian (Rhizoma Coptidis), Huang Qin (Radix Scutellariae Baicalensis) and Bai Mao Gen (Rhizoma Imperatae Cylidricae) for bleeding of nose and gums. Add Da Huang (Radix et Rhizoma Rhei) for constipation or bleeding feces.

Vacuity of Liver and kidney

Manifestations

Purpra that is chronic, repeated attacks, pale color, accompanied with soreness of lower back, five palms hot, night sweating, dizziness and tinnitus, hematuria, red tongue with thin coating, thin and rapid pulse.

Treatment Principle Nourish yin of liver and kidney, invigorate blood.

Formula

Liu Wei Di Huang Wan (Six-ingredient Pill with Rehmannia).

In the formula, Shu Di Huang (Radix Rehmanniae Glutinosae Conquitae) and Shan Zhu Yu (Fructus Corni Officinalis) nourish the kidney and generate liver. Shan Yao (Radix Dioscoreae Oppositae) and Fu Ling (Sclerotium Poria Cocos) strengthen spleen and fill essence. Ze xie (Rhizoma Alismatis Orientalis) and Mu Dan Pi (Cortex Moutan Radicis) clear the liver and stop bleeding. Add Chi Shao (Radix Paeoniae Rubra) Chi Shao (Radix Paeoniae Rubra) and Dan Shen (Radix Salviae Miltiorrhizae) for dark and purple purpura. Add Yin Chai Hu (Radix Stellariae), Di Gu Pi (Cortex Lycii Radicis) and Fu Xiao Mai (Semen Tritici Aestivi Levis) for lower grade fever and night sweating. Add Ju Hua (Flos Chrysanthemi Morifolii) and Shi Jue Ming (Concha Haliotidis) for dizziness and tinnitus.

Lost blood due to qi vacuity

Manifestations

Chronic, recurring attacks, pale and purple purpura, with nose and gums bleeding, pale complexion, poor appetite, palpitation, pale lips and tongue, deep weak pulse.

Treatment Principle Strengthen the spleen and nourish the heart, supplement qi to control blood.

Formula

Gui Pi Tang(Restore the Spleen Decoction)

In the formula, Ren Shen (Radix Ginseng), Huang Qi (Radix Astragali Membranaceus), Dang Gui (Radix Angelicae Sinesis), Zhi Gan Cao (Roasted Licorice Root), Bai Zhu (Rhizoma Atractylodis), Fu Ling (Sclerotium Poria Cocos) augment Qi and blood to control blood. Yuan Zhi (Radix Polygalae Tenuifoliae), Suan Zao Ren (Semen Zizyphi Spinosae), Long Yan Rou (Arillus Euphoriae Longanae) and Fu Ling (Sclerotium Poria Cocos) nourish blood and calm the mind. If there is persistent bleeding, add San Qi (Radix Notoginseng), Pu Huang (Pollen Typhae) and Xue Yu Tan (Crinis Carbonisatus Hominis)

Yang vacuity of the spleen and kidney

Manifestations

Chronic, recurring attacks, pale and purple purpura. There are more on the lower extremities with nose and gums bleeding, lusterless complexion, fatigue, cold extremities, shortness of breath, loose stool, pale tongue with deep weak pulse.

Treatment Principle Warm and tonify the spleen and kidney, nourish essence and blood.

Formula

You Gui Wan (Restore the Right Pill) modified.

In the formula, Shu Di Huang (Radix Rehmanniae Glutinosae Conquitae) and Shan Zhu Yu (Fructus Corni Officinalis) and Gou Qi Z i(Fructus Lycii) nourish kidney essence. Du Zhong (Cortex Eucommiae), Tu Si Zi (Cuscuta Seed), Fu Zi (Radix Aconiti Lateralis Praeparata), Rou Gui (Cortex Cinnamomi Cassiae) and Lu Jiao Jiao (Colla Cornu Cervi) 3-6g replenish the essence and tonify kidney yang. Add Dang Shen (Radix Codonopsitis Pilosulae), Bai Zhu (Rhizoma Atractylodis) and Huang Qi to strengthen qi and control the bleeding. If the purpura occurs repeatedly, add Dan Shen (Radix Salviae Miltiorrhizae) and San Qi (Radix Notoginseng).

Kawasaki's Disease (Chuan Qi Bing 川畸病)

Kawasaki's disease, also known as mucocutaneous lymph node syndrome, is an immune disorder in which the medium-sized blood vessels throughout the body become inflamed manifested with acute fever, injured mucus membranes and swollen lymph nodes. It is largely seen in children less than five years of age. Without treatment, mortality may approach 1%, usually within six weeks of onset. Its rarest but most serious effect is on the heart, where it can cause fatal coronary artery aneurysms in untreated children. In clinic, it is diagnosed and differentiated as a warm pathogen disease as it has acute fever accompanied with rashes.

Etiology and pathology

It is due to an exterior warm pathogen invading the body through the mouth and nose, originating in the Wei to Qi, Ying and Blood levels.

Pathogen in both Wei and Qi level The warm toxin accumulates in the lungs and stomach and enters through the mouth and nose. The lungs control the exterior, the pathogen stays in the lungs, resulting in disharmony of the exterior and Wei, which shows fever and chills. It enters into the interior, and transforms to heat and fire, leading to high fever and thirst due to the heat accumulating in the lungs and stomach.

Flaming of heat in the Qi and Ying level The pathogen from Wei and Qi invades to the Ying level. If the heat toxin mixes with Ying and blood floods to the extremities, it results in reddish toes and fingers. If it stagnates in the neck, it causes swollen lymph nodes of the neck. If the heat toxin is severe, it may injure the vital qi, showing the manifestations of heart yang vacuity, such as pale complexion, purple tongue and palpitations.

Vacuity of both qi and yin Heat toxin lingering inside damages the yin and qi. Because blood flow of the whole body converges in the lungs, Zong qi takes charge of the breath and assists the heart, and manifests as vacuity of qi and yin and will mostly show the symptoms of qi and yin vacuity and blood stasis of the heart.

In summary, Kawasaki's Disease is due to warm heat invading and accumulating in the lungs and stomach through mouth and nose. The heat goes deeper to the Ying and blood level, resulting in flaming of heat in Qi and Ying level. If the heat toxin moves with the blood flow, it involves the heart, or stays inside of the channels and joints, or it can even affect the heart, liver and kidney. The key location of the disease is in lungs and stomach, but it is related to the heart.

Diagnosis

Diagnostic Guidelines

Please refer *Nelson essentials of pediatrics.*

Criteria for Diagnosis of Kawasaki's Disease
Fever of ≥5 days' duration associated with at least four† of these five changes
Bilateral nonsuppurative conjunctivitis
One or more changes of the mucous membranes of the upper respiratory tract, including throat redness, dry cracked lips, red lips, and "strawberry" tongue
One or more changes of the arms and legs, including redness, swelling, skin peeling around the nails, and generalized peeling
Polymorphous rash, primarily truncal
Large lymph nodes in the neck (>1.5 cm in size)

Disease cannot be explained by some other known disease process
A diagnosis of Kawasaki disease can be made if fever and only three changes are present if coronary artery disease is documented by two-dimensionalechocardiography or coronary angiography.
Source: Behrman, Richard E.; Kliegman, Robert; Karen Marcdante; Jenson, Hal B. (2006). *Nelson essentials of pediatrics.* St. Louis, Mo: Elsevier Saunders. <u>ISBN</u> <u>1-4160-0159-X</u>.

Differential Diagnosis

Scarlet Fever The rashes usually appear first on the neck and face (often leaving a clear, unaffected area around the mouth) on the second day after fever starts. It looks like a bad sunburn with tiny bumps. In the body creases, the rash forms the classic red streaks known as Pastia lines. Areas of rash usually turn white when pressed on. By the sixth day of the infection, the rash usually fades, but the affected skin may begin to peel.

Infectious Mononucleosis There is a continuous fever and swollen lymph nodes, but no conjunctivitis or changes in the mucosal membranes of the mouth, no peeled skin on the extremities, WBC count increased to 10 to $20 \times 10^9/L$ or more, Lymphocytes and monocytes increased, more than 50%. Atypical lymphocytes>10%.

Pattern Differentiation

Differentiation guidelines

- Differentiating between the Wei, Qi, Ying and Xue, and distinguishing the depth of the disease. If the disease is at beginning and is in both Wei and Qi, it will invade to the interior and cause heat flaming in Qi and Ying, and even the blood level.
- Differentiate between normal or reversed progression, determine the severity.

Therapeutic principle

Clear heat and expel wind, cool and invigorate blood. Clear heat toxin and expel pathogen from the Ying and Blood to both Wei and Qi. Clear heat, cool and invigorate blood. Supplement qi and nourish for late stage.

Patterns and treatment

Evil in both Wei and Qi levels

Manifestations

Sudden onset, high fever with mild or no chills, thirst, cough with little phlegm, reddish eyes and throat, hot to touch, hard and swollen palms, poor appetite, large lymph nodes in the neck, red tongue with thin white or yellow coating, floating and rapid pulse.

Treatment Principle Expel wind and clear heat with cool and pungent herbs.

Formula

Yin Qiao Bai Hu Tang(Honeysuckle, Forsythia and White Tiger) modified.

In the formula, Yin Qiao San expels wind, clears heat and toxin. Bai Hu Tang clears heat and generates fluid. Add Ban Lan Gen (Radix Isatidis Seu Baphicacanthi), Huang Qin (Radix Scutellariae Baicalensis), She Gan (Belamcanda Chinesis) and Xuan Shen (Radix Scrophulariae Ningpoensis) clear heat.

Heat Flaming in Qi and Ying levels

Manifestations

High fever no subdued, anxiety or drowsiness, rashes, swollen and reddish throat, swollen and painful lymph nodes of neck and behind the ears, reddish palms, dry lips, crimson tongue like a strawberry, purple index vein or thin and rapid pulse.

Treatment Principle

Clear heat and cool the Ying, resolve toxin, cool and invigorate blood.

In the formula, Shui Niu Jiao (Cornu Bubali), Sheng Di Huang (Radix Rehmanniae Glutinosae), Mu Dan Pi (Cortex Moutan Radicis), Xuan Shen (Radix Scrophulariae Ningpoensis) clear heat, nourish Yin, cool and quicken the blood. Huang Lian(Rhizoma Coptidis), Dan Zhu Ye (Herba Loptatheri Gracilis), Jin Yin Hua (Flos Lonicerae Japonicae) and Lian Qiao (Rhizoma Coptidis) clear heat and toxin, expel heat from Ying to Qi.

Concomitant damage to the qi and yin

Manifestations

Fever and rashes have resolved, fatigue, profuse sweating, peeled skin on the extremities, thirst and a desire to drink, red tongue dry coating, purple index vein, or thin and rapid pulse.

Treatment Principle Enrich yin and strengthen qi

Formula

Sheng Mai San (Generate Pulse Powder)

In the formula, Ren Shen (Radix Ginseng) and Mai Men Dong (Tuber Ophiopogonis Japonici) supplement qi and nourish yin, Wu Wei Zi(Fructus Schisandrae Chunensis) astringes the lungs, generates body fluid and stops sweating. Also add Huang Qi (Radix Astragali Membranaceus), Bai Zhu (Rhizoma Atractylodis),Shan Yao (Radix Dioscoreae Oppositae) and Gu Ya (Fructus Oryzae Sativae Germinantus).

If there is a high fever that won't abate, add Zi Xue Dan (Purple Snow Pill), 0.5 pill once a day. M.D. might suggest Aspirin to the patients.

If there are emergent symptoms of the heart, such as myocardial infarction, cardiogenic shock, arrhythmias and heart failure, immediately refer to MD. If in China, TCM might use Sheng Mai Yin (Generate Pulse Liquid), Du Shen Tang (Only Shen Decoction), Shen Fu Tang (Ginseng and Aconiti Decoction), or Sheng Mai Injection (Generate Pulse Injection) intravenous infusion.

Other Therapies

1. Fu Fang Dan Shen Pian (Salviae Co. Pill) taken orally 1 pill, 3 times per day. It is used for blood stasis and increased platelets.

Acupuncture

Evil in both Wei and Qi

Puncture Du14, LI11, St44, SJ5 with purging, no needle retention. Bleeding Lu11 for sore throat. Once a day.

Excessive heat in Qi level

Puncture Du14, LI11, St44, LI4 with purging, no needle retention. Once a day.

Evil in Ying and Blood level

Puncture Ht3, PC8, UB40 and LI11 with purging, no needle retention. Once a day.

Lingering heat with yin vacuity

Puncture Ki3, Ki6, Lu10 and Ren23 with tonifying. If lower grade fever, add SJ6, Du14. If dry throat, add Ren23. Once a day.

Massage

Evil in both Wei and Qi level

Clear lung, calm liver and clear Tian He Shui. If severe fever, add sedate Liu Fu, and lifting Du14.

Lingering heat with yin vacuity

Clear and supplement spleen, knead Er Ma, clear Tian He Shui, push Ki1. If there is lingering fever, add divide Yin and Yang.

Topical therapy

Evil accumulating in Wei level

Grand Chong Bai10g, Dou Chi6g put on the palms for 4 hours once a day.

Heat toxin accumulation

Mix two white part of eggs, honey 30cc, and Da Huang powder 6g, put on the chest 3 hours a day.

Prevention and Care

Etiology of the disease is unknown so far. It may be associated with infection, immune response, environmental pollution, drugs, chemicals, detergents, so there is no specific preventive measure for the cause. In order to prevent myocardial infarction, which is the main cause of death from this disease, it is important to observe the patient every 3~6 months.

Infant and Toddler Eczema
(Ying Er Shi Zhen 婴儿湿疹)

It is also named Nai Xian, a common skin disease in infants and toddlers. It manifests with skin itching and rashes that might look like dry, thickened, scaly skin, or it might be made up of tiny red bumps that ooze or become infected if scratched. Scratching can also cause thickened, darkened, or scarred skin over time. The *Zhu Bing Yuan Hou Lun* (General Treatise on the Causes and Symptoms of diseases) 610 earlier discussed the cause of the disorder "is due to mixed wind with the qi and blood in the skin. ... it is named Nai Xian (milk eczema) due to drinking milk, and the milk stagnates and moves to the face."

Etiology and Pathology

The disorder is most commonly caused by interior damp-heat accumulation mixed with wind, dampness and heat, and shows in the skin.

Congenital weakness and fetal damp heat lingering for an infant If the child is congenitally weak, and the mother desires to have pungent, acrid and dry food or damp-heat invades during pregnancy, the child inherits damp-heat from his mother, which accumulates in the baby's skin and shows as eczema. The *Wai Ke Zheng Zhong* (Orthodox Manual of Surgery) 1617 states "eczema is due to the mother eating over-pungent foods, the father baking food during pregnancy, heat lingering in the infant, which manifests with whole body eczema, secretions, restlessness and severe itching during sleep."

Invasion of wind, dampness and heat The kid's skin is tender, and exterior pathogens easily invade through skin. If the children haven't been covered well or taken off wet diapers, wind, damp and heat invade the body and mix together, stay in the skin, which manifests maculae, blisters, erosion, and itching.

Incorrect diet and nursing can be a trigger since the spleen is insufficient, the spleen and stomach are damaged and fail to transform the nutrition if the diet is incorrect, which leads to food stagnation and turns into damp-heat. Or the incorrect nursing, such as taking a bath with strong irritative soap, or having irritative cloth, may trigger eczema.

Diagnosis

Diagnostic Guidelines

The rash often shows on the face, cubital fossa and popliteal crease. It might look like dry, thickened, scaly skin, or it might be made up of tiny red bumps that ooze or become infected if scratched. Scratching can also cause thickened, darkened, or scarred skin over time.

It is divided into the dry and wet patterns. The wet one manifests with red papules, blisters, erosion and secretion. It is more common in an overweight baby from 1 to 3 months old. The dry one manifests with reddish, dry skin and desquamation. It is more common in slim children older than one year old. The symptoms may be mild or severe. It tends to disappear when the child has fever or diarrhea, but returns again after the diarrhea stops or fever declines. Most children have a family history of asthma.

Differential Diagnosis

Impetigo usually appears as red sores on the face, especially around a child's nose and mouth. The sores burst, develop honey-colored crusts and spread from upper head or face to lower parts of the head.

Diagnostic Notes

- Note the age of the child, season of onset, nutritive state, and if there are any allergies
- Note the body constitution and the course of a disease
- Note the family history of the child

Pattern Differentiation

Differentiation guidelines

- Differentiate between the nature
- Focus on which one is worse between the wind, dampness and heat. If it is wet pattern manifested with red papules, blisters, erosion and secretion, it means all three wind, dampness and heat are worse. If it is the dry one manifested with reddish, dry skin and desquamation, it indicates the wind and heat are worse.

Therapeutic principle

Expel wind, clear heat and eliminate dampness.

Patterns and treatment

Damp-heat accumulation

Manifestations

Overweight, red papules on the face, blisters, erosion and secretion which spread to the head, neck, trunk and extremities, accompanied with fever, anxiety, poor appetite, red tongue with yellow and greasy coating, purple and floating index vein.

Treatment principle Expel wind, clear heat and eliminate dampness

Formula

Xiao Feng Dao Chi San (Expel Wind and Guide Red Decoction)
    In the formula, Huang Lian (Rhizoma Coptidis) and Sheng Di Huang (Radix Rehmanniae Glutinosae) and Jin Yin Hua (Flos Lonicerae Japonicae) clear heat and toxin. Fu Ling (Sclerotium Poria Cocos), Bai Xian Pi (Cortex Dictammi Dasycarpi), Bo He (Herba Menthae Haplocalycis) and Tong Cao (Tetrapanax

Papyriferus) expel wind and eliminate dampness. If the wind is severe, add Chan Tui (Periostracum Cicadae) and Fang Feng (Redix Ledebouriella Divaricatae). If there is severe secretion, add Che Qian Zi (Plantago Asiatica) and Cang Zhu (Rhizoma Atractylodis). if the heat severe, add Lian Qiao (Fructus Forsythiae Suspensae) and Zhi Zi (Fructus Gardeniae Jasminoidis).

Wind-heat lingering

Manifestations

Slim body, recurrently reddish and dry skin, or small red papules and itching, no secretion after scratching, red tongue with less coating, purple index vein.

Treatment principle

Expel wind and clear heat.

Formula

Yin Qiao San (Honeysuckle and Forsythia Powder) modified.

In the formula, Jing Jie (Herbs Seu Flos Schizonepetae Tenuifoliae), Bo He (Herba Menthae Haplocalycis), Dan Dou Chi (Semen Sojae Praeparatum), Jin Yin Hua (Flos Lonicerae Japonicae) and Lian Qiao (Rhizoma Coptidis) clear heat and toxin, expel wind. If there is severe itching, also add Bai Xian Pi (Cortex Dictammi Dasycarpi), Fang Feng (Redix Ledebouriella Divaricatae). If there is dryness and desquamation, add Sha Shen (Radix Adenophorae Strictae) and Mai Men Dong (Tuber Ophiopogonis Japonici).

Other Therapies

Er Miao San (Two Marvel Powder) with sesame topical used for wet pattern of eczema. Zi Cao (Radix Arnebiae Seu Lithospermi) oil topical used for dry pattern of eczema.

Prevention and Care

- Avoid scrubbing the affected area with water and soap. If the scab is thick, it can be moistened with sesame oil first, then gently take off the scab.
- The nursing mother should avoid spicy, fragrant, dry, fishy, duck, beef, lamb and other foods that the child is allergic to.
- Avoid wearing clothes that are wool, or synthetic. Avoid wearing thick clothes. Avoid strong sunlight.
- Try to avoid scratching and rubbing the lesions skin.

ABOUT BAISONG ZHONG

Dr. Baisong Zhong Ph.D, L.Ac, He received his Bachelor of Medicine degree at the Luzhou Medical College (1983), he achieved his Master's degree (1990) after studying with one of China's most famous TCM pediatricians, Professor Xiao Zhengan. He obtained his Ph.D (1997) with Dr. Wu Kangheng, one of the most prominent professors of integrative pediatric and internal medicine at the Chengdu University of Traditional Chinese Medicine, which is the one of the four oldest and most respected Chinese Medical Universities in China. He has practiced, taught and researched in the pediatrics department of the Luzhou Teaching Hospital as well as the Chengdu University of TCM since 1983 until he was invited to American College of Acupuncture and Oriental Medicine(ACAOM) in Houston, TX.

He did research related to five Patent Herbal formulas and medicines, such as Wushan Granules (Patent Herb for removing Blood stasis and reinforcing Qi and Yin.) Sanctioned by State Food and Drug Administration of China (SFDA) in 1999, Terazosin Capsules (Western Medicine for hypertension) Sanctioned by China SFDA.1998, and Fongye Kechuanping liquid (Patent Herb for resolving phlegm and relieve asthma) sanctioned by China SFDA in 1994. He directed and assisted on nine research teams on pediatrics and TCM internal medicine. Examples of these include, A Survey on The Relationship between Children's Physical Constitution and Immunity (1995), Clinical and Experimental Study on Shengyan Capules for Acute Nephritis in Children (1995), and Experimental Study on 'Yiqi Yangyingye' for Children's Diarrhea (2000). He has published the Text Book of Pediatrics of TCM (in Chinese.

It is a text book for TCM university students in China), Test Prep Workbook for the NCCAOM Bio-medicine Module, Test Prep Workbook Test Workbook for Basic TCM Theory in English, and other pediatrics books of TCM. He also published more than 30 papers on modern research related to TCM pediatrics. He is currently a professor and dean of academic clinical training at the American College of Acupuncture and Oriental Medicine (ACAOM), Houston, TX.

Printed in the United States
By Bookmasters